PRAGMATICS

PRAGMATICS
From Theory to Practice

edited by

Judith Felson Duchan

Lynne E. Hewitt

Rae M. Sonnenmeier

State University of New York at Buffalo

PRENTICE HALL, Englewood Cliffs, New Jersey 07632

Library of Congress Cataloging-in-Publication Data

Pragmatics: from theory to practice / edited by Judith Felson Duchan,
  Lynne E. Hewitt, Rae M. Sonnenmeier.
      p. cm.
  Includes bibliographical references and index.
  ISBN 0-13-678988-9
    1. Language disorders in children.   2. Pragmatics.   I. Duchan,
  Judith F.   II. Hewitt, Lynne E.   III. Sonnenmeier, Rae M.
  RJ496.L35P737   1993
  618.92'85ɔ—dc20   93-10009
                                                              CIP

Acquisitions editor: Charlyce Jones Owen
Copy editor: Linda B. Pawelchak
Prepress buyer: Kelly Behr
Manufacturing buyer: Mary Ann Gloriande
Editorial assistant: Nicole Signoretti
Cover design: Violet Lake Studio

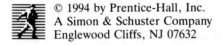 © 1994 by Prentice-Hall, Inc.
A Simon & Schuster Company
Englewood Cliffs, NJ 07632

Printed in the United States of America

10 9 8 7 6 5 4 3 2

ISBN 0-13-678988-9

PRENTICE-HALL INTERNATIONAL (UK) LIMITED, *London*
PRENTICE-HALL OF AUSTRALIA PTY. LIMITED, *Sydney*
PRENTICE-HALL CANADA INC., *Toronto*
PRENTICE-HALL HISPANOAMERICANA, S.A., *Mexico*
PRENTICE-HALL OF INDIA PRIVATE LIMITED, *New Delhi*
PRENTICE-HALL OF JAPAN, INC., *Tokyo*
SIMON & SCHUSTER ASIA PTE. LTD., *Singapore*
EDITORA PRENTICE-HALL DO BRASIL, LTDA., *Rio de Janeiro*

CONTENTS

PREFACE

There are two views of pragmatics in language. The first sees pragmatics as a relatively isolated component of language. The other sees pragmatics as integral to all aspects of language. This latter view necessitates revising most traditional approaches to research and clinical work in language acquisition. It challenges us to maintain a complex, functionally and contextually integrated view of language, and to incorporate it into research and clinical practice.

This book is designed to be consistent with the integrated approach to pragmatics and to advance it by examining its implications for facilitating language development in children with language disorders. The chapters are structured around four commonly occurring contexts for language: conversation, narrative, school events, and familiar home routines. The overall intent of the book is to accelerate the rate at which pragmatics theorizing and practice can become integrated into a coherent framework.

This book is intended for researchers and practitioners as well as for students. While aimed specifically at those in the area of speech–language pathology, its contents will be of interest to educators, special educators, specialists in child language acquisition, developmental psychologists, and anthropologists studying the ethnography of speaking. The book will be of particular relevance in courses covering language teaching methods both in first and second language acquisition as well as language intervention for those with communication disorders.

This book is an outgrowth of a conference held in Buffalo, New York, on March 27 and 28, 1992, entitled Pragmatics: From Theory to Therapy.

The conference was sponsored by the University at Buffalo's Department of Communicative Disorders and Sciences, the Center for Cognitive Science, and a grant from the Conferences in the Disciplines. Invaluable assistance in organizing the conference was provided by Catherine Munroe-Reynolds. The staff of the University at Buffalo's Office of Conference Operations, Bill Regan and Mabel Sumpter, also deserve our thanks for their aid. Finally, we are grateful to the speakers, panelists, and attendees of that conference for creating a stimulating exchange of ideas—an exchange involving discourse across disciplinary boundaries and between academics and practitioners. It is our hope that the lively exchange created at the conference will continue and expand through the readership of this book.

AFFILIATIONS
AND RESEARCH EMPHASES
OF THE CONTRIBUTORS

Bonnie Brinton is an Associate Scientist at the University of Kansas, Parsons Research Center, Bureau of Child Research. Her research emphasis has been on studying development of conversational skills in children and developing assessment and intervention approaches for facilitating conversational skills in children with communication handicaps.

Martha B. Crago teaches and carries out her research in the School of Communication Disorders at McGill University. She has used ethnographic approaches to study Inuit children and adults, with a special focus on how to bring ethnographic methods into the clinical approaches used by speech-language pathologists.

Barbara Culatta is affiliated with the Department of Speech Communication at the University of Rhode Island. Her research has been in the area of language intervention, with a special emphasis on using stories to teach language structure.

David K. Dickinson is affiliated with Clark University, where he carries out research on children's development of literacy skills. His work with Catherine Snow involves aspects of interaction between teachers and children in preschool and elementary school contexts.

Judith Felson Duchan is a professor in the Department of Communicative Disorders and Sciences at the University at Buffalo. Her research emphasis has been on the communication of children with autism. Her current focus is on theoretical and practical implications of the success of facilitated communication with individuals with severe communication disorders.

Alice Eriks-Brophy is a doctoral student in the School of Human Communication Disorders at McGill University. Her research is focused on ethnographic approaches, which she has used in her study of Inuit children.

Martin Fujiki is an Associate Scientist at the University of Kansas, Parsons Research Center, Bureau of Child Research. His research is on conversational abilities of individuals with language disorders and clinical approaches to assessing and facilitating development of conversational skills.

Gail S. Goodman is affiliated with the Department of Psychology at the University of California at Davis. Her research program involves studying the abilities of children to provide eyewitness testimony. Her research emphasis has also been on studying children's memory for schemas, especially event memories.

Lynne E. Hewitt is a speech-language pathologist and a doctoral student at the University at Buffalo in the Department of Communication Disorders and Sciences. Her research has been focused on discourse structuring with a special emphasis on arguments among adults who are mentally retarded, narratives of normally developing children, and the discourse of adults with autism.

Vivian Gussin Paley is a kindergarten teacher at the Laboratory School associated with the University of Chicago. She has published widely on events occurring in her story-based classroom and the many children she has influenced and who have influenced her.

Bambi B. Schieffelin is affiliated with the Department of Anthropology at New York University. Her research focus has been on ethnography of communication among the Kaluli peoples of New Guinea.

Catherine E. Snow is from the Harvard Graduate School of Education. Her early work was on aspects of talk directed by parents to their children. Her recent work is on factors related to children's acquisition of literacy.

Rae M. Sonnenmeier is a speech-language pathologist and a doctoral student in the Department of Communicative Disorders and Sciences at the University at Buffalo. She is studying the interactions of children and adults during the process of facilitated communication. She is also investigating how event knowledge aids language learning in children with language disorders.

Janet Wilde Astington is affiliated with the Institute of Child Study at the University of Toronto. Her research focus has been on the ability of typically developing children to ascribe mental states to others.

chapter 1

THREE THEMES

Stage Two Pragmatics, Combating Marginalization, and the Relation of Theory and Practice

Judith Felson Duchan, Lynne E. Hewitt, Rae M. Sonnenmeier

The children in Vivian Paley's kindergarten classroom tell and enact stories that represent major themes in their lives (Chapter 2). So it is fitting that we find in Paley's chapter the major themes contained in this book. Her story-based classroom epitomizes how language used by children can be situated in a meaningful and exciting event, and how we, as adults in the children's world, can create contexts in which they feel compelled to make themselves understood. The children in Paley's classroom are moved to be coherent by their passion to tell and participate in the enactment of their own and others' stories. From Paley's description of children's story dictation, one gets a sense of how language teaching can be carried out meaningfully and naturally in everyday life events.

Paley describes the marginality that is experienced by some of her children, and the majority's tendency to collaborate in placing these children in the social margin of classroom interactions. She also describes how these dynamics can be reversed under the spell of stories. During story time, children's unusual behavior and ideas become part of the drama. In the context of the story, their aggression is that of a character and is not taken as a direct threat. Children cooperate more during story time so that the story can continue—they put more than one character in their story for Serena, who "panics when a story has only one character" (p. 15).

The chapter written by Paley raises questions about a teacher's stance toward morality in the creation of classroom rules, and about the true nature of narrative as a form of social communication rather than a depiction of the narrator's private thoughts. She concludes about the latter that the child authors in her classroom do not create narratives in social isolation, as did Marcel Proust or Emily Dickinson. Rather, her children's stories are dictated and enacted together, as socially constructed events. Because of Paley's moral leadership, the children on the periphery of her classroom alter the ordinary activities and refocus the rest of the group. The refocusing eventually allows for the "stranger [to become] a fully participating member of the group" (p. 11). Vivian Paley's story of her classroom is a morality tale in which the teacher not only creates an atmosphere for learning and understanding, but also an atmosphere in which children are not allowed to be ostracized.

We use Paley's chapter to set the stage for the remaining chapters in the book. Three themes, found in Paley, are pivotal to the organization and integration of the book:

1. Pragmatics research and teaching methods are ready to be brought to a new level of contextualization, one in which the discourse context and event context are seen as critical to learning language and hence must always be uppermost in our minds as we plan our interventions.
2. Researchers and professionals need to work actively to reverse the forces at work in our culture that lead to the ostracism of children who are different.
3. Theory and practice should be interactive, and engaged in perpetual dialogue, to the enrichment of both.

We now turn to a discussion of the three themes and indicate how they are treated both explicitly and tacitly by the authors of the remaining chapters.

STAGE TWO PRAGMATICS

This book represents and argues for a new evolution in the development of pragmatics. The early pragmatics approach, which could be called **Stage One Pragmatics,** was focused on divorcing itself from two marriages: behaviorism and transformational grammar. The aims of Stage One Pragmatics were to treat learning as more than reinforced stimulus–response associations and to treat language learning as more than an accumulation of linguistic rules (see Craig, 1983; Snow, Midkiff-Borunda, Small, & Proctor, 1984). In addition to saying what it was not, Stage One Pragmatics embraced several components of communicative competence as an expression of what it was. Stage One Pragmatics as incorporated in the practice of speech-language pathology emphasized (1) intents or speech acts, (2) conversational turns, (3) and semantic contingency.

Stage One Pragmatics based intervention programs on finding differences between typical and atypical children's expressions of intent. We borrowed the taxonomies of Dore (1975) and Halliday (1975) to assess children's acquisition of intents, and we developed intervention programs to fill the gaps where they occurred. The focus was that of Bloom and Lahey's 1978 version of "use" in their formulation of form, content, and use as the three basic components of language. Intervention programs were developed to teach children to express requests (Olswang, Kriegsmann, & Mastergeorge, 1982) and to increase their responsiveness to other's requests (Fey, 1986).

A second focus of Stage One Pragmatics was on conversational turn taking. Children were evaluated for their abilities to take turns, and if found deficient, they were provided with intervention programs that helped them learn to take conversational turns. James MacDonald's approaches exemplify this conversational focus (MacDonald, 1989; MacDonald & Gillette, 1984).

Stage One Pragmatics also emphasized the role of the interactant in children's learning of language. The research carried out by Snow (1982) and others (e.g., Cross, 1978) revealed the importance of the input language in children's language learning. In particular, the facilitative role of the adult's immediate response to the child's meaning was emphasized. The principle of semantic contingency led to the development of parent training programs such as Manolsen's Hanen program (Girolometto, Greenberg, & Manolson, 1986). Parents were trained to respond to what children communicated by acknowledging their intent, expanding on their meanings, and recasting their grammatical constructions.

The information in this book builds upon Stage One Pragmatics by creating theoretical and intervention approaches that lead to a **Stage Two Pragmatics.** While Stage One Pragmatics provided intentional and conversational contexts for language learning, Stage Two Pragmatics expands the focus on context to include discourse genres other than conversations and to include the event structure in its theorizing and practice. It still treats requests, conversational turns, and semantic contingency as central, but it considers them as situated in events or discourse genres, rather than as separable from their specific uses.

This situated approach promotes goals in which the linguistic and event context is primary, thereby causing a variety of communicative acts to arise naturally. For example, requesting per se would not be taught; rather, the need to request would be naturally interwoven into a larger event structure. Turn taking would be viewed as being governed by conventions of particular events, rather than as an abstracted skill, separable from the event taking place. Further, a situated approach treats semantic contingency as varying in its effectiveness depending upon how it fits the child's intents, meanings, or understanding of events. Finally, a situated approach would add contexts that were not emphasized under Stage One Pragmatics, expanding our horizons to take in the complexity of real-world communication (see Sonnenmeier, Chapter 10). Of particular importance is the need to acknowledge the varied nature of children's cultural experience, and how these differences are reflected in their language at home and at school (see Crago & Eriks-Brophy, Chapter 4; and Schieffelin, Chapter 3). Unlike Stage One approaches, a situated approach varies its goals and procedures to fit the experiences of particular children in their everyday contexts.

Using a situated, Stage Two Pragmatics approach, professionals can expand their scope of practice beyond their roles as interactants and supply children with contexts to facilitate communication growth. In addition, they can act as advocates, working to change the child's world; as consultants, providing others with ways to facilitate the child's communicative growth; and as ethnographers, developing an understanding of the child in his or her cultural context. This broadening of our scope is a direct reflection of a deepening understanding of language. In this sense, redefinition of our role will increase our effectiveness and improve our productivity.

We have been emphasizing the importance of broadening the definition of context in Stage Two Pragmatics. To help focus our ideas about context, we have selected certain types of situations to explore on this deeper level: **conversations, narratives,** and events taking place at **home and school.** Conversations and narratives are contexts that structure the situation by providing a format for the discourse. Home and school contexts contain familiar events (e.g., bedtime, snack time, sharing time) that structure the interaction and organize the language taking place within them. The four contexts were selected as essential for children to know about, as well as being examples of situations experienced by all children.

The **conversational context** is emphasized in chapters by Schieffelin (Chapter 3), Crago and Eriks-Brophy (Chapter 4), and Brinton and Fujiki (Chapter 5). Schieffelin and Crago and Eriks-Brophy concentrate on the ways adults and children from different cultures converse together, and how these conversations serve to transmit values about interaction and provide contexts for language learning. Schieffelin's revelations about the positive functions of code switching in the conversations between a Haitian child and his relatives bring us to a better understanding of the true nature of bilingualism. Schieffelin argues against previous views emphasizing the necessity for separating the two languages to avoid so-called "language interference." Rather, she shows us how bilingual adults use children's first language understandings to translate and clarify second language use. Crago and Eriks-Brophy, in their study of talk between Inuit children and their older caretakers, found a set of conversational patterns associated with important cultural events and discovered that different family members converse differently with children. Their work eloquently makes the case for the critical importance of culture in language and indicates the risks involved in ignoring children's home language use when planning classroom events.

Brinton and Fujiki show how conversation can be used as a context for teaching children about language structure as well as about components of conversation. They describe their intervention with middle-class American children who have delayed or different conversational skills. Their approach targets three areas: turn taking, topic manipulation, and repair of conversational breakdowns. The authors illustrate their point by describing a preschooler, J, who improved his vocabulary, syntactic complexity, and conversational ability after experiencing an intervention program carried out in a conversational context. Brinton and Fujiki focus, in particular, on the family-based nature of their program, showing how inclusion of J's mother was critical to J's improved communicative competence. This approach exemplifies one means by which contexts for language intervention may be broadened.

Astington provides an interesting bridge between conversational and **narrative contexts** by reviewing the literature on children's ability to take the perspective of another. In both conversations and narratives, children need to learn to organize their discourse to be in accord with their presumed audience's beliefs, feelings, and background knowledge. They therefore need to be mindreaders in that they must develop a theory about their audience's way of thinking. Astington reviews the literature on the stages of development of typical children's theories of others' minds.

Hewitt (Chapter 7) centers on one type of children's mindreading, that involved when they ascribe subjective states to their story characters in the context of reading narratives. Hewitt presents an intervention program that she designed for a teenager who is autistic, to help him better interpret characters' motivations, feelings, and mental states when he reads fictional stories. She argues that one of the merits of emphasizing a character's experience when teaching narrative is that this focus leads us beyond superficial aspects of narrative structure into a living linguistic realm in which fiction offers us revelations impossible in any other form of communication.

Culatta (Chapter 8) also uses narrative as a context for language learning and lays out a detailed approach to language intervention using event and story enactments. She sees narrative as emerging naturally out of the children's role play of daily events. Narratives require different knowledge from that involved in event descriptions or enactments. For narrative understanding children must add to their notions of simple action sequences the notions of blocked goals and complex interrelated events. Culatta's description of motivated goals in narrative understanding provides a complement to Hewitt's discussion in Chapter 7 of how the subjective nature of narrative gives rise to structures, such as goals, that are rooted in characters' experience.

A third context governing language learning, that of **daily routinized events,** is pivotal in chapters by Goodman, Duchan, and Sonnenmeier (Chapter 9), Sonnenmeier (Chapter 10), and Duchan (Chapter 11). As children learn everyday events, they store them as conceptual, integrated schemas (called *scripts*), which they use subsequently to participate in the events, to remember them, and to talk about them. Goodman et al. review the research literature on typical children's learning about events and present a model for studying, assessing, and facilitating children's learning of event representations. Sonnenmeier presents a program for teaching aspects of event knowledge and the language that goes with them. Duchan's chapter discusses intervention principles that might be used with children who are too dependent on scripts—those who have been identified as gestalt learners.

The fourth type of context is that of **preschool classrooms.** Snow (Chapter 12) suggests that in order to become skilled at reading and writing, children must shift from the here-and-now pragmatics of conversational face-to-face interactions to a more distanced pragmatics. She appeals to us to go beyond the linguistic code in helping children achieve literacy, and to include in our practice a way to help children understand the distanced pragmatics of written communication.

Dickinson (Chapter 13) identifies a group of domains in oral language interaction that relate to children's literacy development. He has studied interactions in preschool classrooms and found that teachers and children talk together in a variety of ways, depending on the age of the child, the amount of structure of the activity, whether or not the teacher is roaming around the classroom or remaining stationary, and the teacher's style of interaction. Dickinson also found that the types of interactions between teachers and children in classrooms influence children's later performance on tests measuring academic and language abilities. Dickinson offers suggestions for teaching strategies, derived from his findings about which practices best correlate with literacy.

COMBATING MARGINALIZATION

Besides fostering a shift to situated pragmatics, this book contains ideas about how to avoid marginalizing cultural groups as well as individuals within a culture. In the small culture of her kindergarten classroom, Paley (Chapter 2) has created an atmosphere of acceptance, thus providing her unusual children with dignity and a way of participating within the social group. Under her policy of nonexclusion, Paley's children regard those who are potentially marginal as core members of the class. Schieffelin (Chapter 3) moves us from the culture of the classroom to that of the society, showing how researchers' theorizing has treated cultural groups as marginal by viewing their cultural practices as deviant, undesirable, or unimportant. Using code shifting to illustrate her point, Schieffelin counters negative views toward it. Similarly, Crago and Eriks-Brophy (Chapter 4), by studying the interaction patterns of children and their caretakers, counter contentions that the children's participation in Anglo-based classrooms is deviant. Rather, the children are participating in ways consistent with their culture and it is the classroom style that is deviant and inappropriate. Crago's way of going about studying the Inuit families offers a method for how professionals from a host culture can come to understand the children they work with, and how those same professionals with their new understandings can transform their ways of interacting with the children to be in accord with their cultural patterns. Finally, Duchan (Chapter 11) considers unusual learners, those called gestalt-style learners, who come to understand their world and language in large rather than small conceptual or linguistic units. She makes an appeal for regarding this type of learning as legitimate. She suggests principles for working with gestalt learners with language problems that tailor the language teaching programs to fit the children's understandings and use of specific gestalt forms.

THE RELATIONSHIP BETWEEN THEORY AND PRACTICE

The influences between theory and practice are usually depicted as unidirectional—moving from theory to practice. Indeed, the very title of this book suggests that it will offer a needed translation of current theorizing in pragmatics to educational and clinical practice. The book contains arguments that practice should be sensitive to theorizing, and practitioners should be aware of the theories that motivate the methods in common use. The notion that we are moving to a new type of pragmatics, one that is situated in genres and events, stems from current theorizing that sees behavior as context embedded and takes issue with context "stripped" approaches (Mishler, 1979). Schieffelin (Chapter 3) exemplifies situation-sensitive theorizing in her study of code switching in its discourse and interactional contexts. She points out the inadequacies of some psycholinguistic theorizing about children's language learning, in that it separates children's utterances from their discourse and interactional contexts. Hewitt (Chapter 7) also illustrates the way theory influences practice in her description of how theoretical renditions of narratives lead to different assessment and intervention approaches. Hewitt puts forward a theoretical approach to narrative focusing on children's understanding of subjective states in story characters. Using ideas from the theory, she designs an intervention program to help a teenager with autism understand fiction.

Goodman et al. (Chapter 9) focus on how a theoretical model of children's understanding of scripts can help us in assessing and designing intervention programs for children. They advocate a theory of processing of scriptal knowledge to understand children's learning of scripts. The authors draw from the theory some ideas about how to view problems children have with learning, remembering, and processing event knowledge.

There are many examples in this text and our field about how theories have led to practice. But what about the other direction of influence, in which practice promotes new theorizing or alters existing theories? Paley (Chapter 2) provides us with a sense of how this might occur. Her approach shows us the wisdom of letting the children reveal to us where the truly important issues lie. Sonnenmeier (Chapter 10) also uses practice to inform theory. She offers a depiction of phases in her design of a method to help children develop event knowledge, in which her theorizing first influenced her practice and her practice then led her to further theorizing.

As this book is being written, we are experiencing the results of a new therapy method, *facilitated communication*. This method involves a facilitator supporting a child's hand, arm, or shoulder as the child spells ideas out on a picture board or alphabet board (Biklen, 1990; Biklen & Crossley, 1992; Crossley, 1992; Crossley & McDonald, 1980). It has brought startling breakthroughs for communicating with autistic children, as well as children with other severe communication and physical disabilities. There are no current theories that would explain this unusual success. Indeed, there is a widespread disbelief in its success because the current theories cannot explain it (Schopler, 1992). We now are met with a practice that has no theory to explain why it works and are left with many theories that explain autism and other communicative disorders in ways that are shown to be wrong. For example, our current views tie communication problems of autistic children to their cognitive disabilities—a view that no longer holds for those who are now able to tell us about their frustrations at being treated as "retarded." We are in the interesting position of having to construct a new theory because of the unexplained success of a particular practice.

CONCLUSION

One of the distinguishing features of this book is its variety. We offer this overview as a means by which the common themes and concerns of our contributors may be read. As understanding of language and communication deepens and broadens, so our scope of inquiry and application expands to encompass new areas offering new insight into old problems. Ultimately, Stage Two Pragmatics is a challenge to all of us working with children to strive to bring our own experience with and intuitions about language and learning into focus, and to remake our theories and practice in the mold of our own best ideas.

REFERENCES

Biklen, D. (1990). Communication unbound: Autism and praxis. *Harvard Educational Review, 60,* 291–314.

Biklen, D., & Crossley, R. (Eds.). (1992). Facilitated communication: Implications for people with autism and other developmental disabilities. *Topics in Language Disorders, 12.*

Bloom, L., & Lahey, M. (1978). *Language development and language disorders.* New York: Wiley.

Craig, H. (1983). Applications of pragmatic language models for intervention. In T. Gallagher & C. Prutting (Eds.), *Pragmatic assessment and intervention issues in language* (pp. 101–127). San Diego, CA: College-Hill Press.

Cross, T. (1978). Mother's speech and its association with rate of linguistic development in young children. In N. Waterson & C. Snow (Eds.), *The development of communication.* New York: Wiley.

Crossley, R. (1992). Lending a hand: A personal account of the development of facilitated communication training. *American Journal of Speech-Language Pathology, 1*(3), 15–18.

Crossley, R., & McDonald, A. (1980). *Anne's coming out.* New York: Penguin.

Dore, J. (1975). Holophrases, speech acts, and language universals. *Journal of Child Language, 2,* 21–40.

Fey, M. (1986). *Language intervention with young children.* San Diego, CA: College-Hill Press.

Girolometto, L., Greenberg, J., & Manolson, A. (1986). Developing dialogue skills: The Hanen early language parent program. *Seminars in Speech and Language, 7,* 367–382.

Halliday, M. (1975). *Learning how to mean: Explorations in the development of language.* London: Edward Arnold.

MacDonald, J. (1989). *Becoming partners with children: From play to conversation.* San Antonio, TX: Special Press.

MacDonald, J., & Gillette, Y. (1984). Conversational engineering. In J. McLean & L. Snyder-McLean (Eds.), *Seminars in Speech and Language, 5,* 171–183.

Mishler, E. (1979). Meaning in context: Is there any other kind? *Harvard Educational Review, 49,* 1–19.

Olswang, L., Kriegsmann, E., & Mastergeorge, A. (1982). Facilitating functional requesting in pragmatically impaired children. *Language Speech and Hearing Services in Schools, 13,* 202–222.

Schopler, E. (1992). Television interview, Canadian National television.

Snow, C. (1982). Are parents language teachers? In K. Borman (Ed.), *The social life of children in a changing society.* Hillsdale, NJ: Lawrence Erlbaum.

Snow, C., Midkiff-Borunda, S., Small, A., & Proctor, A. (1984). Therapy as social interaction: Analyzing the contexts for language remediation. *Topics in Language Disorders, 4,* 72–85.

chapter 2

EVERY CHILD A STORYTELLER

Vivian Gussin Paley

In his novel *The Guermantes Way,* Marcel Proust observes, "Ideas are goddesses who deign at times to make themselves visible to a solitary mortal at a turning in the road . . . but as soon as a companion joins him they vanish. In the society of his fellows no man has ever beheld them."

Thus spake the aloof Proust. Yet what may be true for the mature artist and philosopher can never be so for a child. Ideas are indeed the goddesses Proust imagined and children do behold them in private fantasies. But then it is essential to transfer the ideas to dramatic scenes witnessed and rightfully entered into by others if these ideas are to take wing and fly.

When we are young, ideas come to us in the form of stories, lavishly endowed with characters and plots, and further explained as we play them out with the help of companions. Even the abstract and lyrical visions of the adult Proust surely must have had their beginnings in childhood as he placed himself inside little fantasy worlds that reached their zenith when communicated to others.

Emily Dickinson is another great writer whose inner world flourished in relative isolation. Writing to a friend who sent a letter in common to Emily and her sister Vinnie, the poet cautioned, "A mutual plum is not a plum. I was too respectful to take the pulp and do not like the stone. Send no union letters. The soul must go by Death alone, so, it must by life, if it is a soul. If a committee—no matter" (Higgens, 1967, p. 15).

This too is not the way of children, for whom a mutual plum is far sweeter. That which is heard and acted upon in the company of peers provides the greater confirmation that the soul is not alone and abandoned.

Yet these profound thinkers give awareness to the universe found in each individual. We recognize Proust's "solitary mortal at a turning" and Dickinson's soul that goes by death and life alone. They goad us to search for clues to every child's inner self—as well as to our own—lest we all be swallowed up by the crowd.

However, I want another literary mentor for my classroom, someone who assures us that the individual is part of a society in which each person's story is connected to all the others—Jane Austen, for example. In her novels and letters, the meaning of life waits at the crossroads; she and her characters are bidden to explore a variety of pathways with their fellow creatures, all the while mapping out their own particular detours.

I may feel Proustian at faculty meetings, devoutly wishing everyone would stop talking and let me think, but Austen offers a better metaphor for the classroom. In her gentried parlors, as in our schoolrooms, it is invariably the odd person out, the character who speaks and acts in unexpected and confounding ways, who causes a refocusing of group consciousness. The stranger, newly arrived at the gates, bringing unfamiliar rules and rituals in his wake, ultimately reveals the strengths and flaws of a tight little community.

It is, in fact, only when the stories of these uniquely different outsiders are heard and understood that the community can climb to the next rung of the moral ladder. The process by which the stranger becomes a fully participating member of the group is Austen's morality tale and is the one we must act out in our classrooms as well.

Dylan, Mary Ellen, and Serena are significantly different from the 22 other children in my kindergarten, and from each other. But they share three characteristics in common: a deep distrust of teacher-led activities, a degree of self-absorption beyond the norm, and a varying inability to speak in coherent and familiar ways under ordinary circumstances. To the extent that these three children are able to "be unto us as the homeborn among us," paraphrasing Leviticus, can we call our schoolroom a moral society.

Dylan, to begin with, is the youngest child of college professors. At five, he has not mastered a language or appropriate social behavior. "Me'en a tiger," he growls, pouncing on Shelly, who sits quietly listening to the book I am reading.

"Stop it, Dylan, I'm telling," she snaps, and he slinks away mumbling, "Her deader." He passes but barely notices Mary Ellen scowling at him from the edge of the rug. "Who cares? I isn't listening to you," she hisses, raising her hand threateningly. Nor is she listening to me or the book. Mary Ellen rises to her feet and sashays around the room according to some adult image she copies, stopping when she approaches Serena, the third member of our wandering trio who always leave the group when a book is being read. Serena is at a corner table, writing. She knows how to read and write but takes little pleasure in books or people.

Even so, it is to Serena that Mary Ellen has confided, "My mommy and daddy don't live any more with me." Mary Ellen has been sexually abused and lives now with her grandmother. Her grammar poses no particular problem but she cannot keep unwanted memories, in the form of disconnected words and phrases, out of her sentences for very long.

Serena speaks perfectly but stores her memories in verbal rituals and compulsive behaviors. Her thoughts seem to be controlled by secret codes and categories she invents anew each day. While I read to the class, Serena prints messages on squares of colored paper. Her parents, who own a restaurant, were proud of their daughter's early accomplishments but are now concerned about the strange uses to which she puts her talents.

Before lunch, Serena passes out her neatly printed cards. They read: "NOT-LIBBY," "NOT-ADRIANNE," "NOT-PETER," and so on. We have all been alphabetized and organized by color into nonpersons. A–E is on red, F–J on pink, K–O on white, P–T on blue, and U–Z on yellow. For letters with no corresponding names she has written "R is absent," "Q is absent," "Y is absent," "Z is absent." Her spelling and math are exemplary, but her imagery and social vision are sadly confusing.

The children scratch out "not" when they discover what it says, and Serena screams, "Don't *do* that!" She cries for several minutes, demanding of me, "Tell them not to!" When I explain that the children don't want to be a "not," she is genuinely surprised. "Why don't they?" she asks.

It is tempting to label and classify these three children, much as Serena puts our names on lists governed by a changing set of attributes. She uses her lists and card collections to communicate with us but they seem random and willful. By comparison, our categories seem scientific and purposeful. However, none of the lists, hers or ours, has anything to say about storytelling.

If we listen to the stories that Dylan, Mary Ellen, and Serena tell, we are surprised at what we hear. All three, being so quick to misconstrue the meaning of ordinary events and so frequently involved in puzzling exchanges, are, in fact, passionate and sensible storytellers. They want their stories to be understood and are gratefully cooperative when given the opportunity to act in someone else's story.

Fortunately, storytelling and acting are the mainstay of our curriculum. No matter what other activities we carry out—and this includes a good sampling of the ways we learn to know ourselves and solve our problems—the common ground upon which we build our classroom culture is found in our stories, dictated and acted out each day.

Imagine, if you will, Dylan, Mary Ellen, and Serena at the round table we call the story table. Except at lunch, it is the only place these three are likely to meet voluntarily for a common purpose. The logistics are simple: If you wish to tell a story, which will be acted out at some point during the day, you write your name on the story list. This is the best understood list we have. Dylan finished learning to write his name in order to put it on the list. Mary Ellen, who prints her name beautifully but refuses to identify any product with her name, makes certain it is on the story list before she hangs up her coat in the morning.

Even Serena is so cognizant of the reality of this particular order of names that she often rewrites the list so she can be first. The children object, of course, so she uses the rewritten form for her own purposes and follows the official list for storytelling. She awaits her turn now, fashioning her own private catalogue in which the first and last letter of each name is omitted but then placed into other names according to a complex mathematical design.

Mary Ellen is poised to speak. Hers is usually the most difficult story for me to write down because she begins by inserting material she does not want. She must rid herself of the bad stuff if the good stuff is to emerge: "Once upon a time there was a little puppy—no, he's not going to be in it— just me. And once upon a time there was a big huge wolf says—"

Dylan interrupts, "Red little riding girl?"

"No, it's not," replies Mary Ellen.

Dylan tries again, "A fox is it?"

"He don't know what I'm talking about. Hello? I say hello little pretty." She begins swishing around behind her chair murmuring hello in a sexy voice. There is no other way to describe her voice at such times. "Hello? Hello? I don't have no business. But I *do* have some business." She sounds angry now and Serena responds to the anger by attempting to take control of the sentence.

"No business, some business, any business, all the business, no business," Serena croons. Her chanting and printing often cover all the possible ways of saying something.

"No more 'bout my business!" orders Mary Ellen. "The wolf says I never had a girlfriend before. And I never either had a girlfriend. That's what I say. Don't write that. Girlfriend don't s'posed to be a man. That's not how you do my story. You gotta erasing this."

I follow her instructions. "What does the wolf say?" I ask.

"The wolf part is out. He don't know my business. I want a kitty instead of a wolf. A little cat and a little puppy. No wolf! No boyfriend! No business!" She looks around at all of us as if we are somehow at fault. Then she visibly relaxes and continues in a softer voice, the one she uses when she is ready to tell her "real" story. "And I'm a little girl. And then once upon a time there was a little puppy and a little cat and me. I'm a princess. I'm so lovely."

"Mousie there is?" Dylan asks, and Mary Ellen correctly interprets his question as "Does the girl have a mouse?" She smiles at him. "Yeah, there's a mouse too. We have three pets. Wait, that's not all. So we together, we have a friendship. We *together* saw a rainbow. Then we said, 'Lovely. We want a rainbow in the sky.' Then the mama she said, 'We don't have no time, honey.' " The last sentence is spoken in hushed tones, as if she is remembering something pleasant.

Serena looks at Mary Ellen, then leans over and places her finger on the word "honey" while she reads Mary Ellen's story to herself, probably to determine which words were erased. These events are of great importance to Serena. In her own stories there must be no extra spaces between letters or words, or unintended dots or smudges, no unfinished lines or omitted "ands" and "buts." The children know that Serena anxiously monitors the words that begin and end each sentence.

It is Serena's turn. "Once upon a time there was a yellow jacket. And it stung everything it saw. But one time it accidentally stung a pencil. And one time it accidentally stung a building. And then a little kid came along and it stung the little kid." Serena stops, contorting her face. "Not 'the,' " she whines. "I said 'a,' not 'the.' Why did you write 'the'? Erase that!" She watches to make certain that every sign of the offending word is gone.

"Mine got erased too," Mary Ellen says. "Mine got the wolf erased."

"And the boyfriend and the no business and the girlfriend," Serena says matter-of-factly.

"And the fox," Dylan adds.

"There wasn't no fox, silly! Don't you know nothing, boy?" she shouts good naturedly. Dylan is happy. He is part of a real conversation. This is the longest he'll pay attention to a connected series of events during the school day. He remains at the table until he tells his own story, drawing pictures in his notebook and commenting regularly, a sort of call and response in which he seems to be practicing conversational skills.

Serena continues. "And then his mommy and daddy came and said, 'Why is that little boy crying?' And the yellow jacket stung almost everything in the whole world. And then the mommy and daddy with the little kid were lost. And they lived happily ever after."

Lisa has joined the group at the story table. "It can't be happily," she argues. "If they're lost. You have to find them." But Serena doesn't respond. Lisa's logic, which is our common understanding of these matters, makes no sense to Serena.

As if to prove her point, Lisa tells a story in which only good things happen. "Once upon a time there was a little house and it was waiting for people to move inside. And the the little house was happy. Then the parents had kids and they bought a pet rabbit and then they feeded the pet rabbit every day and then the pet rabbit had babies. The parents let the children take out one of the baby bunnies. And they lived happily ever after."

Lisa's story seems uncomplicated. There are no stinging yellow jackets, no wolves who want little girls for girlfriends, no boyfriends sneaking into a little girl's story, and no family that stays lost forever. The house, family, kids, pets, and babies intend no harm. Yet, when we act out Serena's story, Lisa begs to be the yellow jacket. Almost everyone wants to be the yellow jacket.

Before Dylan tells his story, he warns Serena that no one else will be in it. "Only me. Just fox is me only that." He is preparing her for what he knows she will do: run away from the table. Serena panics when a story has only one character. She has made a number of compromises for the sake of storytelling but she cannot accept a single-character story any more than an empty space on a line, or an unfinished sentence at the bottom of a page. An extra chair at her table or around the story rug must be removed or explained to her satisfaction if she is to stay.

In a one-character story it may seem to Serena that the other characters are absent, and the absentee is a daily source of stress for her. She often singsongs children's names who are *present*, saying they are absent, while claiming the absent ones are present. The children think she is teasing and tell her to stop but we know she won't stop until a certain number of names have been called out.

Dylan's story is brief so Serena doesn't have to stay away long. "Once upon a time come a fox. That me. Growl! Jumping on the hill. And I make my teeth like this. And then running around. Look how strong the fox." He shows me his muscles and then puts a finger on an "and," while whispering Serena's name.

"Speaking of Serena," I whisper back, "do you want to add another character? So when we act out your story, Serena won't cry and run away."

He considers the option for a moment but then shakes his head. Later in the year, he and all the others will methodically avoid one-character stories. In her own stories Serena sometimes tests herself by reducing the number of characters to two. Mary Ellen understands that a struggle is taking place. "You almost down to one, Serena," she says.

Mary Ellen has her own battles. "Once upon a time we was really scary," she dictates one day. "We was pimples and everything. We don't know what to do. We was so frightening. The people was so scared of my separation. And then you say, kiss, kiss, come on, give me a kiss." This time she doesn't ask me to erase anything, and when we act out her story, the chldren are unusually still, watching the actors huddled together on the square of rug we call a stage. Serena is there too, pretending to be frightened. It is a moving experience. Later, in the doll corner, I hear Joanna say to Mary Ellen, "Are you scary? Or are you a baby kitty?"

Mary Ellen begins to purr softly, but the gentle moment vanishes when Dylan grabs Joanna's doll and repeatedly bangs its head on the stove. The characters in his stories do not behave so irrationally. Which is the real Dylan? Both, of course, but in storytelling and acting he is able to pull certain concepts together and focus upon a higher standard of behavior.

The telling and acting out of one's own story is a euphoric experience: self-initiated, self-fulfilling, and self-revealing. It is intensely concentrated and leads to a rewarding act of concentration. Storytelling is of play, from play, about play, and ultimately, the essence of play. It is play under control, a compromise between the solitary soul and the outside culture.

More often than play itself, these stories offer the opportunity for an awkward child to influence the rest of us in positive ways. Dylan, who pounces on people and draws fire, and who says things we cannot always understand, makes sense of himself—and to himself—in his stories. His story language and behavior are well above his ordinary conversation and social interactions.

"Once there was two little bunnies," he begins shortly after the doll-smashing episode. "And then they play. They was eating apples. The bad guy falls them out. Then fox bite the bad guy. Then fox is a friend. He plays with those bunnies even when the dark is here."

Dylan, as storyteller and actor, is more stable, connected, and gracefully literate than during any other school activity. So are Mary Ellen and Serena. This does not surprise me. The more different or difficult a child appears, the more eager and able the child is to use stories as a pathway to the outside world.

Serena puts children at a distance when she signs their names to mysterious, coded lists. But her stories help restore the children's confidence and somehow explain what she is doing at other times.

Here is a story of hers that creates such a bridge:

> Once upon a time there was a school of kids but there was only five kids in the school. Number 1 liked to jump, number 2 liked to play, number 3 liked to build things, number 4 liked to draw, and number 5 liked to be the leader. One day number 5 was the leader but the teacher said number 1 couldn't jump. And then number 5 told number 2 not to play. And then when he was getting the milk, he told number 3 not to build, and when number 5 was going to music, the teacher told number 4 not to draw. And number 5 was the only lucky one that day.

Serena's story reminds me—and perhaps the children also—of something that happened the day before. She refused to help at cleanup time but instead made a list of those who should clean up each day. She then went around informing people of their special day: "*You* cleanup on Wednesday, *you* do it on Friday," she kept on, while the children continued to put things away, barely paying attention to her. The story she has just told helps me understand, in a less emotional context, her great need to control everything in a world in which she controls very little. She spells out—in exaggerated form—feelings the children recognize.

How does storytelling accomplish its task of explaining the individual to the group and the group culture to the individual? There is no mystery here; no convoluted interpretation is required. We are born to be storytellers. From the beginning it is the way we think, the way we analyze our feelings and integrate new ideas.

Even before kindergarten we are prepared to listen to stories and read between their lines. We know how to fill in the spaces and finish the sentences; we can seat the characters on the empty chairs, so to speak, and add the "ands" and "buts." Notice how easily Serena's vernacular aids me in explaining my ideas. Her confusing behavior finds logical expression in her stories and we, the audience, bring to them an emotional background and linguistic context that often fails us elsewhere.

There is no other classroom activity in which such empathy and common knowledge is instantly established. It matters not where we come from or what confusions or developmental lags accompany our entrance into school. The story format includes us all. Even those with minimal language or social skills, who may need to listen for a long while before their own stories emerge, *know* what is going on. It is not very different from what happens in their own minds, though they cannot speak the words that match the pictures.

Now I come to another part of my morality tale. Dylan, Mary Ellen, and Serena are not popular children. Many of these children with exceptional problems are unloved or ignored in school. So indeed are many children *without* serious problems but who seem different or awkward in look or manner. They are also shunned and easily left out of play and other areas that are governed by free social choice.

However, because story is our common heritage and universal learning tool, we must all be given the equal opportunity to tell our stories and participate in those of our classmates. Children must not be allowed to exclude others from any aspect of classroom life in which linguistic, cognitive, and social skills are practiced and improved. In so doing we allow children to limit the learning potential of others and, ultimately, of course, of themselves.

This requires a classroom culture in which no one can say "You can't play." Play is the progenitor of storytelling and is the common property of every child. Play is not only for those who already know how to play and who fit the profile requirements of the group.

For years I have searched for logical reasons to impose certain moral imperatives: You can't say you can't play; you can't choose certain people but not others to be in your play and stories; you may not exclude a single child from any part of the common culture. Morality aside, what are the inherent educational justifications for placing such matters of fairness above friendship and free choice?

The answers come to me as I study those who appear different. These are the children who speak and think and act in unexpected or disconcerting ways, for whom equal access to play and storytelling may be the lifeblood of future development. These are the children who define our responsibilities as a school society; their stories must be heard by everyone.

Dylan, Mary Ellen, and Serena often spoil the play. Dylan's fantasies intrude in physical ways and his contorted explanations frequently miss the mark. "They didn't I haven't in the way because they don't," he tells us, and we don't know what he means.

Mary Ellen's anger is even more of an unwanted imposition. Her suggestive images are harder to deal with than a growling, doll-banging, verb-twisting tiger. Her "So what! I gotta boyfriend. Kiss, kiss, oh, you so pretty!" stops us in our tracks.

And even clawing tigers and scary boyfriends are relatively easy to distract and dissemble compared to Serena's system of private checks and balances that make catastrophic events out of ordinary flexible routines.

Yet we can come together as storytellers while Dylan, Mary Ellen, and Serena are learning to be story players. Somehow, the child who may not evolve naturally as a player is given a second chance to investigate the technique if he or she can tell stories and have them taken seriously by the entire group.

The logic and language of social and linguistic development are found in dramatic episodes. Here is the proper stage for those cognitive questions that need ballast and substance not found in workbooks or diagnostic tests: What does this word mean (so we can act it out)? What does this sentence mean (so we can act it out)? What do these characters say to each other (so we can act them out)?

If you want us to know your story you must slow down and speak the words so that I am able to write them down. If your desire is to have the group act out your story (and it is universally so), then you can't pounce, or keep erasing, or disguise your ideas inside a private code all the time.

Dylan, Mary Ellen, and Serena are no different from the rest of us. They want their story to receive attention. But attention when given in negative ways does not produce satisfaction. Unlike Proust's solitary thinker, the child must step to the rhythm of the group. The imagination is not a unilateral function. It thrives in the company of those who understand its point of view and ask the right questions.

"No fair!" says Eddie to Serena when "kid number 5" gets to have all the fun and make all the decisions. "No fair!" say the others, though they enjoy being in her story. What does "no fair" mean? This is the largest issue on our classroom stage and in the outside world as well.

Those who are different appear not so different after all when their stories are played out. Their stories join the common story bank as we expand our mutual perspectives and learn to relish the sweetness of our mutual plum.

In Serena's story, kid number 5 takes the pulp, while numbers 1, 2, 3, and 4 are left with the stone. Is this the way our classrooms appear to those who remain on the outside? If so, then the plum will surely turn sour, for kid number 5 wishes to be a leader but his tight little society has no solid moral base.

"Wait a minute," says a fifth grade boy whom I quote in my book *You Can't Say You Can't Play* (Paley, 1992). "In your whole life you're not going to go through life never being excluded, so you may as well learn it now." The speaker has the look of someone who has known rejection. He is overweight and pimply and has a slight stutter. "Kids are going to get in the habit of thinking they're not going to be excluded so much with your new rule and it isn't true."

"Maybe our classrooms can be nicer than the outside world," I say, while he shakes his head. "But this way you won't get down on yourself when you do get excluded," he tells me.

It is difficult to refute the argument of this awkward and intense 10-year-old. "Okay," I continue, "but as a teacher, here's what troubles me. Too often it's the same children, year after year, who bear the burden of rejection. They're made to feel like strangers."

Well, perhaps this is what school is all about. We enter each new classroom as strangers and some among us seem destined to remain strangers. Must this always be so? There is much for us to ponder as we continue our study of children's lives in the classroom. We will not make a mistake if we focus the group's attention upon those in need and encourage them to tell us their stories. They are the ones who help explain what we are doing in school.

REFERENCES

Higgens, D. (1967). *Portrait of Emily Dickinson*. New Brunswick, NJ: Rutgers University Press.

Paley, V. Gussin. (1992). *You Can't Say You Can't Play*. Cambridge, MA: Harvard University Press.

Proust, M. *The Guermantes Way* (Part 11).

chapter 3

CODE-SWITCHING AND LANGUAGE SOCIALIZATION
Some Probable Relationships
Bambi B. Schieffelin

INTRODUCTION

In this chapter I explore some probable relationships between code-switching and general processes of language socialization. Several research paradigms, each with different goals and methodologies, have focused on young children's bilingual language use in an attempt to answer a variety of psycholinguistic and sociolinguistic questions. Code-switching, which is the use of two different languages and/or dialects (codes) by the same speaker within the same speech situation or conversation, plays many important functions in speech communities all over the world (Gumperz, 1967, 1982). The majority of the research in this area has been carried out with adult speakers and among school-aged children, usually in peer settings, usually by sociolinguists. The aims of this research include understanding the syntactic constraints that organize code-switches and the possible social meanings of different types of switches. Code-switching in terms of the role it plays in the acquisition of language(s) has not been explored.

The study of language socialization, which shares many concerns with developmental pragmatics and language acquisition, is grounded in ethnographic studies of language use (Ochs & Schieffelin, 1984; Schieffelin & Ochs,

1986b). It focuses on socialization *through the use of language* and socialization *to use language*. A basic assumption of this perspective is that for all children, the acquisition of language entails the acquisition of critical aspects of cultural knowledge, including information about social relationships, values, and ways of acquiring knowledge. Language socialization studies have been carried out in a number of Western and non-Western societies; however, the speech communities that have received the most attention have been monolingual (Schieffelin & Ochs, 1986a, 1986b; but see Kulick, 1992).

In this chapter, a brief review of relevant literature in early bilingual language acquisition is followed by selected literature on children's code-switching to illustrate how the formulation of research questions in each area has generated particular findings. One of the major gaps concerns the nature of the verbal environment of bilingual children and its role in understanding what children say and how they say it. I outline some of the reasons why bilingual language acquisition and code-switching should be studied in an integrative manner, and I suggest that language socialization is the best framework for accomplishing this. Drawing on data from language socialization research in several Haitian Kreyòl/English–speaking households in New York, I show how conversations in which participants use more than one language provide excellent opportunities to study the transmission and acquisition of cultural and linguistic knowledge. We can see what adult and child speakers know and what linguistic resources they draw on when talking to each other. Thus, ethnographic and sociolinguistic perspectives can not only lend insight into cultural practices, but can also be informative for psycholinguistic research as well.

Like most research in social science and the humanities, scientific inquiry on language acquisition is deeply affected by cultural, linguistic, and socio-economic ideologies held by both researchers and their subjects. Such cultural and linguistic ideologies are often associated with political and social attitudes that involve values assigned to the variety of language spoken ("prestige form," "nonstandard dialects"), and to particular languages themselves as being more or less prestigious. These attitudes are never limited to language itself but are extended to the speakers of particular languages and language varieties. These ideologies, often unexamined, strongly affect the object of study, the research methods used, the type of research questions asked, the type of data collected (and not collected), and who is studied. Furthermore, these ideologies influence the ways in which data are interpreted.

The literature on child bilingualism is a rich area in which to explore some of these underlying attitudes because bilingual situations are not only linguistically complex, but socially, culturally, and politically complicated as well (Gal, 1987; Grosjean, 1982; Hamers & Blanc, 1989; Romaine, 1989). Research on bilingualism is disciplinarily broad, covering a range of formal and informal learning contexts and the life span (Hyltenstam & Obler, 1989).

My interest, however, is in pre–school-age children growing up in bilingual (and multilingual) environments who learn two or more languages in non-school settings. These children are learning language(s) during what Genesee calls the primary language learning years (1–5) (Genesee, 1989).

CONTRIBUTIONS FROM DEVELOPMENTAL PSYCHOLINGUISTICS TO CHILD BILINGUALISM

The early studies of infant bilingual acquisition in the first half of this century were taken up with debates as to whether or not the acquisition of more than one language was in fact detrimental to the child's intellectual, social, and emotional development (see Diaz, 1985; Hakuta, 1986; and Weinreich, 1953, for different views of this issue). Questions are still raised about the benefits of bilingual acquisition in contemporary psycholinguistic research. Studies of bilingual middle-class families living in monolingual speech communities in Europe, Australia, or the United States have been carried out in which one parent spoke a "minority" language and the other spoke the majority language.[1] Psycholinguistic studies in different Spanish/English bilingual speech communities in the United States have taken up similar issues. In addition, there have been an increasing number of sociolinguistic studies of these same bilingual communities (and others) that have added new theoretical dimensions to the acquisition process and provided important insights into adult and child language practices.[2] The results of these different types of studies have been used to argue about benefits and disadvantages of particular bilingual practices in terms of the child's linguistic development and to evaluate bilingual policies in the schools.

Although bi- and multilingual development research shares many theoretical and methodological concerns with studies of monolingual children, there are some questions that have been highlighted in first language acquisition but are notably missing in bilingual acquisition. The most striking is the way input has been studied. Many researchers in first language acquisition study the nature and role of input directly, through audio and videotape recordings of caregiver–child interaction. Although there are diverse opinions regarding the *role* of input, as a result of empirical research we have an informed idea of its linguistic and sociolinguistic *nature* in many different speech communities (Schieffelin & Ochs, 1986a, 1986b; Snow & Ferguson, 1977). This has not been the case in most studies of early bilingual acquisition; and with very few exceptions, input has not been studied directly (de Houwer, 1990; Genesee, 1989; Goodz, 1989).

Early diary studies (Leopold 1939–1949; Ronjat, 1913) and later psycholinguistic experiments in the 1970s and 1980s centered on simultaneous bilingual acquisition. They asked if children acquire two independent language systems at the outset, or whether they acquire one that is gradually distinguished. The assumption in many of these studies was that if children were presented with two linguistic codes, each should be clearly differentiated. This could be in terms of parental usage (one parent = one language, "Grammont's Rule"), particular settings, or both. The presence or absence of a child's language mixing or mixed utterances ("interference") was taken as evidence to support different arguments regarding the nature of the acquisition process in terms of the separateness of the two codes. The child's psycholinguistic development was established through analyses of child speech production data. With more than one language used in the verbal environment, this type of research focused on the interaction between the two systems at the levels of phonology, vocabulary, and syntax. The questions focused on whether bilinguals acquire their two languages in much the same way as monolinguals, particularly in terms of *rate* of acquisition and *order* of syntactic structures acquired.

Studies that focused on bilingual acquisition include Padilla and Liebman (1975), Padilla and Lindholm (1976), and Lindholm and Padilla (1978). Their research designs had several things in common. Data consisted of audiotaped interactions between young bilingual (Spanish/English) children in different American speech communities in California and the Southwest. Data on the verbal environments of these children were provided only by parental report; there was no direct investigation of speech to the child by the parents or others involved in child care. In order to evaluate the child's ability to speak each language, Padilla and Lindholm (1976) and Lindholm and Padilla (1978) had each child interact separately with two experimenters, each of whom spoke to the child in only one language. Only firstborn children were studied so as not to complicate the acquisition picture with input from siblings. Conversations between experimenter and child are not reported. Code-switching, which is an important linguistic resource in several of the communities studied, is not discussed. Clearly, a highly selective view of the bilingual child's verbal environment was the object of study.

In contrast to psycholinguistic studies of children growing up in established bilingual speech communities, there exists a set of studies of bilingual families who are not members of such speech communities. Although there may not be preferred community norms, it is likely that there are individual styles of code-switching in these families when speaking to or in front of young children. Volterra and Taeschner (1978), for example, investigated stages of bilingual acquisition of two children in a family context in Rome where each parent spoke only one language to the child (Italian/German). Based on tape recordings in alternate language environments, child production data were analyzed in terms of various syntactic constructions as they appeared in both languages. Of interest to these two authors was the issue of interference when the child was in "situations of conflict," that is, interacting with people speaking different languages. The authors claim that children learned rules to "minimize the risk of interference" (Volterra & Taeschner, 1978, p. 325) to reduce the language production effort. Over time, the tendency to label people with definite languages decreases, and the child accepts the possibility of speaking either of two languages with the same person. From their perspective, being truly bilingual is viewed as "speaking both languages fluently with any person." While this type of bilingualism may be appropriate in some communities, it is not the case in others where particular codes are reserved for particular addressees, even if both speaker and addressee are bilingual. Only limited discourse data are presented, and there is no mention of code-switching.

A similar study of bilingual acquisition in German-speaking families was carried out by Redlinger and Park (1980). They observed four firstborn children at different developmental stages over a period ranging from five to nine months. For the taped speech samples collected in children's homes, experimenter Redlinger spoke only or primarily German, and the mother spoke in the other language (Spanish/English/French). Language usage in the home was again limited to self-report and mothers estimated percentages of first and second languages that they spoke to the child. Some mothers claimed that each person only used one language, but others claimed that while both languages were used "children were not exposed to language mixing within sentence boundaries" (Redlinger & Park, 1980, p. 338).

Concerned with the question of language mixing in relation to linguistic development, Redlinger and Park concluded that children whose language was more advanced (measured by Mean Length of Utterance excluding mixed utterances) produced fewer mixed utterances than the children at earlier stages of development, suggesting that the amount of mixing and language development is inversely associated (1980, p. 340). The lack of strict language separation was seen to have an effect on the high rate of mixing by one child, whose mother reported speaking an estimated 70 percent Spanish and 30 percent German. High mixing rates on the part of the child are interpreted as the child's inability to differentiate between two languages. The child to whom speech was reportedly separated by speaker had the least mixing. In an analysis of structural types of mixtures found in the corpus, child sentences are listed without the discourse context or sequence in which they were produced. Redlinger and Park support the proposal that single system processing gradually shifts to two systems, supporting the findings by Volterra and Taeschner (1978).

Other researchers have studied the rate of syntactic development and vocabulary growth in bilingual children by comparing families who maintain a parent/language separation and families in which both parents spoke both languages. Doyle, Champagne, and Segalowitz (1978) found no difference in the linguistic performance of the two groups of children. It should be pointed out that the parent's language was not studied directly; authors relied on parent-reported usage via telephone interview.

The question of whether children who are simultaneously acquiring two languages initially go through a stage of linguistic production when the two languages are mixed ("linguistic confusion") or whether they have a unitary undifferentiated language system is taken up in an unusually clear manner by Genesee (1989), who examines the various explanations of "mixing" during early bilingual development. He also calls for greater attention to the study of parental input in addressing these questions.

The issues raised in these and many other psycholinguistic studies of bilingual language acquisition concern the nature of the child's knowledge of the linguistic codes, how these codes are acquired, and the relationship between the codes. Here we can locate some of the ideological underpinnings of this work. Implicit in this body of literature is the idea that monolingual acquisition is the "norm" and learning a second language is potentially problematic. McLaughlin (1981) suggests that keeping the codes separate either by speaker or setting helps the child to keep the two languages separate. The more language mixing in persons and places, the more the developmental pattern is likely to diverge from typical monolingual patterns. McLaughlin (1984) goes on to suggest that

> the optimal conditions for minimizing language mixing occur when both languages are spoken consistently in the home by different persons. When the languages are mixed by adult speakers, or when one language becomes dominant, one finds more mixing in the child's speech. If one language is spoken in the home and the second is acquired through acquaintances, playmates, balance seems to be upset and more mixing occurs. (p. 27)

Given this view, it is no surprise that the majority of bilingual acquisition studies have selected parents who claim to use only one language in speaking to the child and focus on firstborns to avoid the complexities of input from other sources.

This leads to two problems. First, it assumes that one needs only to consider parent input, a view that makes particular assumptions about family and household composition and the social organization of caregiving. Second, since the focus is on child speech, many take on faith what parents report, or they do not report what parents actually say. They also assume that what parents say about their input is accurate. However, as Gumperz has pointed out, code choice and code-switching are often done out of the awareness of speakers. To ask a bilingual to report on switched forms is like asking a monolingual to report instances of using the future tense (1982, p. 62). Self-report information, although interesting in terms of attitudes, cannot be equated with actual speech practices.

This point is beautifully illustrated by Goodz's (1989) longitudinal study of French/English–speaking families in Quebec, which included an analysis of the linguistic input to four firstborn children where one parent was a native English speaker and the other a native French speaker. All parents declared themselves to be firmly committed to speaking only their native language when addressing their children (p. 29). What Goodz found was that parental ideology and parental report did not match parental practice, a finding that is not surprising to sociolinguists or linguistic anthropologists. She found that at least some mixing or switching occurred during all parent–child interactions. Although the frequency of child language mixing was relatively low, Goodz had strong evidence that language mixing, especially for mother–child dyads, is closely related in terms of discourse (1989, p. 38).[3]

To ignore input in any and all forms not only skews the research questions but makes interpretation of data extremely ambiguous. The psycholinguistic literature on bilingual acquisition (including Hakuta's important book) fails to include input, including code-switching as a conversational practice. Multilingual speech practices are complicated to study, but like other culturally organized activities they can and must be empirically investigated. As Kulick (1992) has pointed out, multilingual input can have surprising consequences, including the loss of the vernacular. He reminds us that the fluid and "mixed" input that children growing up in bi- and multilingual communities receive is more common than the one-person/one-language strategy that exists in a relatively small number of households.

From much of what has been written in the psycholinguistic literature, we can infer a particular linguistic ideology about bilingualism. Bilingualism is viewed as a set of abstract structures in the mind of the individual, not as a set of cultural and linguistic practices displayed between speakers. A "balanced bilingualism," the ability to speak any language to any person, is preferred, a view of language use and language distribution that is counter to the preferences and practices in many speech communities. Additional assumptions in the psycholinguistic literature are that code separation both in the mind and in speech practices is desirable and that patterns of monolingual acquisition are the basic model.

Furthermore, code mixing is not encouraged as a learning strategy. McLaughlin states that

> the conditions of language presentation have important consequences for language differentiation. Attaining bilingual competence is more difficult the more mixing the child is exposed to, although it seems likely that mixed exposure does not lead to permanent retardation in either language. In fact researchers sometimes mistake mixing in the child's speech for confusion and language interference, when the child is actually using or trying to use mixed utterances rhetorically for sociolinguistic purposes, just as adult speakers in the child's linguistic environment do. (1984, p. 27)

Even though McLaughlin clearly acknowledges the possibility that children might use "mixed utterances" for sociolinguistic purposes, this aspect of language use has yet to be systematically pursued by those doing psycholinguistic research on young child bilinguals.

To summarize, with the rare exception, the study of bilingual acquisition has not included the direct investigation of the input of parents and relevant others. In addition, the research paradigm has implicit assumptions about the nature and value of bilingualism, code-switching, and the nature of language itself. These assumptions have led to the stigmatizing of code-switching as language confusion.

THE PERSPECTIVE FROM SOCIOLINGUISTICS ON CHILDREN'S CODE-SWITCHING

While psycholinguists in the mid-1970s and 1980s were investigating the extent to which different language codes could be kept separate by young bilingual speakers, sociolinguists took as their starting point not languages, but speech communities with cultural preferences for using language and languages in a variety of ways (Gumperz & Hymes, 1972). This perspective took a stance different from the Chomskyian view of language favored by the psycholinguists, which was seeing language primarily as an abstract grammatical system. In contrast, language was viewed by the sociolinguists as a symbolic system capable of carrying affective, social, and pragmatic as well as referential information. Sociolinguists faced the complex problem of investigating the heterogeneity of spoken language as presented by speech registers, dialects, and multiple languages and speech varieties. Starting in the 1960s, researchers such as Ferguson, Fishman, Gumperz, Labov, Hymes, and others set critical research agendas and devised various linguistic and ethnographic methods for investigating how meaning is conveyed through variation at the phonological, lexical, grammatical, and pragmatic levels of language. These ideas gave further support to the notion that language is more than a system of abstract rules in one person's mind; rather, it is a system of communicative conventions shared by members of speech communities and it is used to establish, maintain, and organize social life.

One of the most challenging forms of speech behavior documented by sociolinguists is conversational code-switching, the use of alternative languages or dialects to express social meaning within the same turn of speaking or utterance (Blom & Gumperz, 1972). Both in some scientific and lay speech communities, code-switching has been viewed negatively, a sign of "laziness or sloppiness of speech," evidence of a deficit on the part of a speaker in one or two languages. Terms such as *semilingual* suggest incompetence, and *interference, impure,* and *mixed* suggest contamination. Sociolinguists, who are interested in the attitudes speakers have toward such complex communicative behaviors, have studied the systematic patterning of code-switching practices in a range of speech communities both within and outside the United States (Gumperz, 1982; Heller, 1988; Kulick, 1992; Poplack, 1981; Zentella, 1990, among many others).

Initial interest in the acquisition of children's code-switching strategies developed as part of a commitment to investigate the development of communicative competence of nonmainstream children growing up in bi- and multilingual speech communities in the United States. Most of this work has focused on bilingual Spanish/English–speaking communities (Duran, 1981; Keller, Teschner, & Viera, 1976). More recently, attention has focused on language use, including code-switching, among European children who migrate with their families who are seeking improved economic situations (see, for example, Auer, 1988).

I will briefly compare selected psycholinguistic studies of child bilingualism with several major sociolinguistic studies of bilingual children's speech practices in order to highlight similarities and differences in methods and theories. Genishi (1981), McClure (1977), and Zentella (1981) were among the leaders in sociolinguistic studies of children's code-switching. All carried out field research in large Spanish/English bilingual communities in different parts of the United States. The study of educational settings and peer conversations from children over four years of age were among the features shared across their research projects. Data consisted of children's tape-recorded conversations with a variety of participants. Based on analyses of spontaneous conversations, these analysts detailed the verbal strategies used by children with peers or researchers and compared the functions of code-switching among child peers to what has been described for adults within the child's speech community. A consistent finding across these and other studies is that children's alternation between languages is neither random nor the result of a linguistic deficit. As with adult speakers, social, grammatical and functional principles govern these children's code-switches. Their ability to code-switch identifies them as members of particular communities and represents a skillful use of language for social or stylistic ends.

Sociolinguistic studies on children's code-switching were similar in method and theoretical perspective to work by Fillmore (1976) and Ervin-Tripp (1981) on children's second language acquisition. Both sets of research focused on children's verbal strategies, emphasizing the kinds of social and linguistic knowledge (conversational knowledge) children bring to the task of acquiring another language. However, like psycholinguistic studies of bilingual acquisition, research on children's code-switching tended to neglect the study of young children's acquisition of code-switching in conversation within a family context and thus did not contribute to our understanding of the role or nature of input to children's language learning in bilingual speech communities.

Even though there have been a few studies that have focused on adult–child interaction, the discourse itself has not been considered as part of the context to be investigated. For example, in her study of a three-generational bilingual Spanish/English family in El Paso, Texas, Huertas-Macias (1981) classified code-switching utterances by form or grammatical class and looked at speech functions in the conversations between adult family members who spoke Spanish at home but also employed code-switching in approximately one-third of their utterances. She also examined the speech of one child (25–34 months) being raised in this bilingual environment who was acquiring both Spanish and English. However, she presents the child's code-switching in terms of its utterance distribution, out of its discourse context, so one cannot tell how talk to the child was organized or how code-switching was used. In this respect, her work resembles the psycholinguistic studies.

Garcia (1980) collected longitudinal tape recordings of 12 bilingual Spanish/English mother–child dyads (ages ranging between 28–32 months at the start of the study) in preschool settings in Utah and investigated interactions in which conversational code-switching was used. He found that mothers rarely code-switched, but when they did, it was for two major functions. The first he labeled *instruction*—where information about one language was given in the other or instructions were given about language use. The second he called *translation*—where the same information was given in both languages. Garcia suggested that although code-switching is infrequent it had a very meaningful functional relationship to conversational clarification "and possibly language learning (teaching)" (p. 243). Moreover, using code-switching, mothers were taking an active role in language teaching. Looking at the examples Garcia presented, these two functions, instruction and translation, seem to be widely used in language learning contexts.

Methodology, however, is often an issue when examining studies comparatively because there are disagreements about what constitutes a switch, the boundary of a switch, and the status of particular words in particular speech communities in terms of their assignment to one or another code (see McClure 1977, 1981, Zentella, 1990, for comprehensive and insightful perspectives on this issue). As Zentella (1990) points out, beyond methodological issues there remains the problem of comparability across speech communities since the linguistic function and social meaning of code-switching varies across bilingual speech communities. She suggests that one must take a broader view of the social distribution of patterns, the organization of speech activities in terms of the ways in which languages are used, and the analysis of exchanges between bilingual adults and children across a range of settings. Further, the attitudes concerning the choice of codes and code-switching, as well as the awareness of the choice of codes and code-switching, must be adequately investigated before political and educational decisions are made about their acceptance. This position differs from the more universalistic approaches to psycholinguistic aspects of bilingual acquisition.

Thus, with few exceptions, the developmental psycho- and sociolinguistic literatures have not focused on the verbal environment of young children learning more than one language. Questions remain unanswered as to how patterns of code-switching are acquired by children, and how code-switching is related to processes of language acquisition.

LANGUAGE SOCIALIZATION: AN INTEGRATIVE
THEORETICAL FRAMEWORK

Language socialization, socialization *through* the use of language and socialization *to use* language, provides an integrative theoretical framework in which
to consider such complex linguistic behaviors as code-switching and other
aspects of multilingual language use. For all children, acquiring language
entails acquiring critical aspects of their culture, ideas about relationships,
values, and methods for acquiring knowledge (Boggs, 1985; Clancy, 1986;
Crago, 1988; Crago & Eriks-Brophy, Chapter 4; Heath, 1983; Kulick, 1992;
Miller, 1982; Miller, Potts, Fung, Hoogstra, & Mintz, 1990; Ochs, 1988; Schieffelin, 1990; Watson-Gegeo & Gegeo, 1986, among others). Generally, studying the acquisition of cultural and linguistic knowledge in any population adds
to our understanding of general learning processes and specific cultural
preferences.

One of the first requirements in a language socialization study is to
identify important contexts and activities of socialization and the participants
who organize them. In most parts of the world the household is a major site
for socializing activities and the members of the household are important
participants in those activities. It is within this context that one can determine
the social organization of caregiving, attitudes and assumptions about teaching
and learning, and the status and role of the child in that particular society.
An important dimension of early socialization is the fact that caregivers display
appropriate attitudes toward other speakers and toward language—which one
to speak, when to speak, how to speak. Studying language in "natural contexts" is essential because it is in these situations that caregivers display
their socializing techniques and children are able to demonstrate their competence.

Research on verbal interaction across cultures has demonstrated that
discourse is a critical resource for understanding what participants are doing
when they interact. Discourse is not merely a sequence of utterances, but a
displayed set of norms, preferences, and expectations relating discourse structures to context, which speakers draw on and modify in producing and interpreting language in context (Ochs, 1988). For example, analyses of
misunderstanding and clarification sequences can be very illuminating about
local theories of the person, and of ideas about intentionality. By participating
in such sequences children are socialized into culturally specific ideas about
not being understood (Ochs, 1990). They learn verbal and nonverbal strategies
for solving those problems. Experiencing misunderstanding provides children
with the foundation for constructing interpretative frameworks and developing
hypotheses about the nature of ambiguity. Work on clarification requests,
repair, and paraphrase (for example, Cherry, 1979; Garvey, 1977; Golinkoff,
1983; Ochs, 1990; Snow, 1977) has demonstrated the willingness of white
middle-class American caregivers to guess, expand, and offer a range of verbal

hypotheses to the child who has not made him- or herself clear. In contrast, ethnographic research in other communities, for example Kaluli and Samoan, show different ways of responding to children's unintelligible or indeterminate utterances. These adults prefer their language equivalents of "huh? what?" and do not offer explicit verbal guesses (Ochs & Schieffelin, 1984). These preferences socialize the child into very different worldviews about solving the problem of not being understood, specifically who is expected to provide verbal responses and what kind. In Kaluli and Samoan society, this work is largely left to young language learners; they are responsible for reformulating utterances and making themselves understood. Therefore, with regard to the larger discourse level, we can ask: How are children socialized into displaying that they do not know something, or do not know how to say something? What types of solutions are offered by caregivers to these problems, and what roles do different languages play in accomplishing this?

It is well established that all children learn language in the context of dialogue and social interaction with more knowledgeable members of their social group. In addition, we know from work in conversation analysis (led by Sacks, Schegloff, & Jefferson) that understanding between participants in an interaction must be achieved through joint attention and intersubjectivity, often on a turn-by-turn basis (see review in Goodwin & Heritage, 1990). Therefore when studying language socialization one must ask questions about how dialogue is constructed (dyadic, multiparty) and organized by local social orders, local theories of knowledge, communication, and competence; how comprehension is acknowledged and noncomprehension repaired in conversation (Schegloff, Jefferson and Sacks, 1977); and how adults and children manage miscommunication when they have more than one code available to them.

Misunderstanding is an important problem-solving activity with which all participants in interaction must deal. Solutions to misunderstandings are culturally organized according to local ideologies and beliefs about learning and language use (Ochs, 1990). In multilingual communities that use code-switching in everyday conversation, code-switching can serve as an important means of repairing as well as facilitating conversation, in addition to being an important resource in establishing social identities.

There may be particular advantages in using code-switching in dialogues with young language learners. For example, code-switching can be viewed as a way to facilitate comprehension; a means to achieve dialogic interaction; a route to language learning; a way to enhance metalinguistic awareness; a method for "learning how to learn," what Bateson (1972) calls deutero-learning; a way of socializing multiple cultural identities; and a way of acquiring more than one language (but it is also a way in which children can learn to be monolingual, cf. Kulick, 1992).

In summary, three questions that have theoretical and methodological implications can be posed:

1. From a psycholinguistic perspective: What is the nature and role of input in the verbal environment of bilingual or multilingual children? What is the range of variation?

2. From a sociolinguistic perspective: What role might code-switching in discourse play in language development and language socialization?

3. In families and speech communities that regularly code-switch as part of their verbal repertoire: How is code-switching as a speech style acquired? Is code-switching between adults and children structurally and pragmatically similar to adult speech practices?

CODE-SWITCHING IN A HAITIAN FAMILY

The questions that I have been raising grew out of a pilot project on language socialization in Haitian Kreyòl-speaking families living in New York City. Haitians rank as the fourth largest group of new immigrants in this city, and estimates put their numbers at over half a million individuals. The latest report (1989) from the Coordination Committee on Haitian Affairs indicates that Haitian students constitute the third largest language minority attending New York City public schools. There has been no research on language socialization in Kreyòl-speaking families in Haiti or any Haitian diaspora community. Over the course of eight months I tape-recorded the spontaneously occurring verbal activities of five young children in several households and the people with whom they regularly interacted. This included, in addition to their mothers, their fathers, aunts, uncles, grandparents, babysitters, cousins, and family friends. Variations in family migration patterns, social class, education, family structure and organization, and social networks contribute to the heterogenity of the Haitian community. Different residential and personal histories have contributed to the fact that Haitians have different linguistic repertoires. In many ways these children typify the linguistic and social heterogeneity found in Haitian diaspora communities in New York City. Because of this heterogeneity, one cannot generalize about "all Haitian children."

The verbal environments of Haitian children in New York City are varied in terms of languages spoken. Parental input may be predominately Kreyòl, or it may include standard or other varieties of English, Spanish, and/or French to varying degrees. Other relatives, such as older siblings, are actively involved in social interaction with small children; and many households include several generations, all of whom may have different linguistic preferences. Children are also cared for by babysitters, many of whom are monolingual Kreyòl speakers. Television provides English to greater or lesser extents. For many Haitians, the Kreyòl language is a critical part of their social identity; it is not linked to literacy and schooling, nor is it taught in formal contexts. Most Haitians in New York City assume that their children will learn Kreyòl.

The examples I have selected focus on one child, Yves, who, in addition to his parents, regularly spends time with his paternal grandparents, cousins, aunts, and uncles. Most of his extended family members are multilingual—some speak mostly Kreyòl, others speak more English, French is rarely used. Yves arrived in New York from Haiti at two years of age speaking only Kreyòl. With his parents he joined the household of his paternal grandparents who, like many other Haitians, came to New York in the mid-1960s and raised their children here. Just before Yves reached his third birthday I began audiotaping him while taking detailed contextual notes; the tapes were transcribed and annotated with the assistance of native Kreyòl speakers. Yves was very eager to speak English and took the opportunity to use it with his aunt who was fluent in Kreyòl and English. He usually spoke Kreyòl with his mother, who understood some English but did not usually speak it with him. The transcripts of these spontaneous family interactions represent a range of adult–child and child–child activities, from dyads to more complex interactional arrangements. In this family, code-switching frequently occurs in conversations between adults, between adults and children, and between children (cousins).

As we will see in the examples that follow, Kreyòl/English code-switching is a resource not only for learning conversational skills, but for Yves it is a way to acquire a second language. Yves deploys code-switching to elicit translations, explanations, and clarifications. In these examples, and throughout the transcripts generally, code-switching between Yves and his multilingual aunt was used to translate between the two languages and instruct particular usage, similar to the functions described by Garcia (1980) for Spanish/English bilinguals. This pattern of code-switching seems particular to this adult–child dyad and is different from the ways in which Yves's aunt code-switches with multilingual adults. These patterns of use can be viewed as part of a speech register for language learning signaled by particular code-switching functions (Schieffelin, in prep.). As will be seen, the majority of Kreyòl/English code-switches occur between utterances (intersentential), but there are also many examples of within-sentence switches (intrasentential) produced by both adult and child speakers.

The examples that follow are taken from two two-hour samples of Yves's speech collected when he was 3 years, 4 months. They show how alternating between the two languages is a way of solving communication problems related to gaps in knowledge of word meaning, grammatical structure, and cultural knowledge. Kreyòl is underlined and glosses are provided.[4]

1. Yves (Y) at home with his mother (M), infant brother, and aunt (A).

    (Y is making car noises as he runs around)
1 M   Yves! sa w'ap fè bwi konsa? m'ap mete ou chita wi.
    [Yves! *why are you making noise like that? I'm going to make you sit down.*]
2 Y   (loudly) what? I said what!
3 A   what are you doing now?
4 Y   I'm doing now.

 5 A yea.
 6 Y I'm doing—/
 7 A w'ap fè kisa?
       [*what are you doing?*]
 8 Y —/ like this.
 9 A m'pa konprann non cheri. di m' an Kreyòl kisa w'ap fè la.
       [*I don't understand dear. tell me in Kreyòl what you are doing.*]
10 Y kisa m'ap fè la?:
       [*what am I doing?*]
11 A yea kou ou ta fè konsa ((sounds)) kisa sa ye?
       [*when were you doing like that ((sounds)) what is that?*]
12 Y non paseu m' t'ap gade t'vizyon like this.
       [*no because I was watching television* like this]
13 M li t'ap gade televizyon like this.
       [*he was watching television* like this.]
14 A oh, I see. oh ou t'ap gade televizyon like this? oh, se egzersis ou t'ap fè? kèu
       ou wè nan televizyon?
       [oh, I see. oh *you were watching television* like this? oh, *is it exercises that you
       were doing? that you saw on television?*]

Yves' mother, worried that he will disturb his infant brother, addresses him
in Kreyòl, the language she usually uses with him. He responds to her in
English with a repair initiator, 'what? I said what!', which he says when he
doesn't like what she has just said to him (2Y). His aunt joins in, in English
(3A). Yves responds to his aunt in English but does not provide adequate
information (4Y–6Y) so his aunt code-switches to Kreyòl in an attempt to
facilitate communication (7A), asking him 'what are you doing?', a translation of her English utterance (3A). Yves answers in English but is treated
as not understood, and his aunt responds to him in Kreyòl (9A) with an
other-initiated repair, 'I don't understand dear. Tell me in Kreyòl what
you are doing.' She makes explicit the fact that she does not understand
him (the problem) and then tells him to speak Kreyòl (the solution), another example of both instruction and translation. He responds in Kreyòl
(10Y) and she then asks more specifically about the sounds he was making
(11A). His answer is 'no because I was watching television like this' (12Y).
His mother paraphrases his Kreyòl utterance (shifting to third person) and
repeats the intrasentential code-switched English phrase 'like this' (13M), and
his aunt starts her answer to him in English, but switches to Kreyòl, paraphrasing what he has said including the English phrase 'like this', and adds
'was it exercises that you're doing? That you saw on television?' Thus code-
switching is presented as a way to achieve understanding. When Yves and his
mother are alone, their conversations are in Kreyòl, but when his aunt is
present he will sometimes use English in response to his mother's attempts
to control his behavior, which often draws his aunt into the conversation. By
investigating the range of usual participants (beyond parents), we see another
view of language use.

2. Yves with his aunt (A) and his cousin (1.6) having a snack.

1 Y   —/I don't want this. (re: muffin)
2 A   what <u>toutou</u>?
3 Y   don't want this.
4 A   what <u>chouchou</u>?
5 Y   I don't want this. I don't want this.
6 A   <u>di m' an Kreyòl</u>.
      [*tell me in Kreyòl*]
7 Y   I don't want this. I don't want this.
8 A   you don't want this? <u>ou pa vle l' ankò</u>? okay, <u>ou pa bezwen manje l'depoze</u>
      <u>l', si ou pa vle/si ou pa vle manje l'depoze l'</u>.
      [*you don't want this? you don't want this? okay, you don't want to eat it, put*
      it down, if you don't want/if you don't want to eat it, put it down]
9 Y   <u>m' pa vle manje ankò</u>.
      [*I don't want to eat it anymore*]
10 A okay, <u>men w'ap manje sa a</u>? okay. okay <u>fin manje ti mòso sa a pou ou ka bwè</u>
      <u>ju</u>.
      [okay, *but you will eat that?* okay. okay *finish eating that little piece there and*
      you can drink some juice]
11 Y I don't want juice.
12 A you don't want juice? I'll just leave the juice here, okay? if you guys want
      some more you can help yourself. okay? I'll leave it on the table.

Throughout her conversations, whether she is speaking Kreyòl or English, Yves's aunt only uses Kreyòl terms of affection (<u>toutou</u>, <u>chouchou</u>, lines 2A, 4A) with him and her own child. After several failed attempts to understand what Yves is saying in English about his muffin (2A, 4A), his aunt initiates a switch to Kreyòl and offers him a possible solution to the problem she is having understanding what he is saying (6A) 'tell me in Kreyòl.' She tells him to use the language he knows best, an example of the instruction function on language use, but he continues in English. She evidences her understanding by her clarification query of what he has said (8A), first in English and she then translates it into Kreyòl, an example of the translation function of code-switching. His response in Kreyòl (9Y) 'I don't want to eat it anymore' is followed by her other-initiated repair in Kreyòl which she confirms herself (okay). She also offers him juice (10A) which he rejects (11Y), switching to English to answer. Her next turn maintains his language choice. Both adult and child speakers initiate code-switches during their conversation, and both within and across turns use code-switching to paraphrase or repeat what they have just said, or the other has said. The next example illustrates both the instruction and translation functions to which code-switching is put.

3. Later that day, Yves is playing with a little figure, aunt (A) and cousin (1.6) watch.

1 Y   this is ((play sounds))—/horse. ((play sounds)) like this. (Y picks up little man
      figure)

2 A what—that's a sheriff? how do you know that's a sheriff?
3 Y this is ti tonton not sheriff. I said ti tonton here.
     [this is *little man* not sheriff. I said *little man* here.]
4 A oh se ti tonton?
     [oh, *it's a little man?*]
5 Y wi!
     [*yes!*]
6 A okay. what do you call a ti tonton in English?
7 Y yes.
8 A how do you call a ti tonton in English?
9 Y —/in English?
10 A enhen. Ki jan ou rele ti tonton an angle?
     [*uh huh. how do you call a* ti tonton *in English?*]
11 Y (loudly, running around)—/a rabbit!—/
12 A that's not, that's not how they call the ti tonton in English, do you know? You
     can say you don't know.
13 Y I don't know.
14 A you don't know? okay, I'll tell you. Ti tonton sa-[*this little man*]
15 Y wi-[*yes*]
16 A okay, oh nou ka rele l' a little man.
     [okay, oh *we call it* a little man]
17 Y (excitedly jumping up and down) oh a little man! yes a little man! yes!

In this example, Yves responds to his aunt's query about the name of the
small figure in an utterance that contains both English and Kreyòl elements.
He emphasizes what he has said (3Y) ('I said') and when his aunt questions
him about the name, she switches to Kreyòl (4A) 'oh se ti tonton', to which
Yves responds in Kreyòl 'yes'. The next lines illustrate the instruction function
as his aunt asks him if he knows the English word for ti tonton (6A) and this
time he answers her English utterance in English. But when she asks him for
the translation and he cannot answer (9Y) she herself translates the request
made in 8A to Kreyòl (10A). This answer fits within both translation and
instruction functions which in these data are often found together. It is clear
from the sequence (8A–12A) that he does not know, and what is important
in terms of language socialization is that his aunt having switched back to
English tells him what to say when he doesn't know (12A), another example
of instruction on language use (13Y). Her next lines use both languages and
we see how Yves follows her lead in code-switching, responding in Kreyòl
after a Kreyòl phrase (14A–15Y), but switching to English after the English
phrase (16A–17Y). Here we see a query in one language about another (10A)
(instruction) and a strategy is displayed for solving the problem of finding out
a word meaning: use both languages. After being told what the English word
is, Yves uses it immediately, and also throughout the afternoon.

Two other observations about this example: one is the extensive use of
verbs of saying in both languages: 'said', 'call', 'rele', 'say', 'tell', showing the
pervasiveness of talk about talk, enhancing metalinguistic usage and awareness
in both languages. Another observation concerns the use of pronouns that

co-occur with these verbs. The shifting reveals subtle choices of stance and identification with the languages that are being spoken and spoken about. After realizing that Yves does not know the equivalent term in English for ti tonton, his aunt says (12A) 'that's not how they call' meaning those that speak English, but when speaking Kreyòl (16A) she uses nou ka rele, 'we call', identifying themselves as Kreyòl speakers.

The final example shows more of the established pattern of code-switching used between participants in these family conversations and the amount of talk around negotiating and achieving meaning, in both languages.

4. Y at his house with mother, infant brother, and aunt

1 Y nennenn kot Eddy en?
 [*nennenn where is Eddy?*]
2 A mwen di w' deja, cheri, Eddy is home
 [*I told you already, dear,* Eddy is home]
3 Y Eddy is home
4 A yea Eddy is at home. Eddy's sick
5 Y sick. what sick?
6 A what sick?—malad
 [what sick?—*sick*]
7 Y malad. what malad? kote l' malad? kote l' malad?
 [*sick.* what *sick? where is he sick? where is he sick*]
8 A kote l' malad?
 [*where is he sick?*]
9 Y wi
 [*yes*]
10 A li li gen—gripe, yea li gen gripe
 [*he he has—flu,* yea *he has flu*]
11 Y kote l' kote l' malad en?
 [*where is he, where is he sick?*]
12 M li gripe Yves! li grip Yves!
 [*he has the flu Yves! he has the flu Yves!*]
13 Y mwen konnen!
 [*I know!*]
14 M oh w'ap mande kote l' malad? li gripe Yves!
 [*did you ask where he is sick? he has the flu*]

In this sequence Yves asks his aunt (whom he addresses as 'nennenn') about his cousin. She responds in Kreyòl 'I told you already, dear' then she shifts to English—'Eddy is home'. Yves repeats this English utterance (3Y) and it is again said by his aunt (4A) who adds that Eddy is sick. Yves questions this (5Y) and his aunt, repeating what he has said 'where is he sick?', is not sure whether he understands the English word 'sick' or whether he is asking about what kind of sickness. She provides the Kreyòl word for 'sick'. But Yves wants to know where (which part of the body) and shifts between Kreyòl and English to ask (7Y). Lines 8A–9Y concern establishing that that is in fact what he wants to know. His aunt, continuing in Kreyòl (10A) tells him that 'he has flu' but Yves continues to ask the same question (11Y), to which his mother essentially says what his aunt has already told him, to which he loudly responds 'I know!' (13Y). This elicits an annoyed response from his mother 'did you ask where he is sick?', again calling attention to the talk itself.

One of the things we can see in all of these examples is that Yves is learning techniques about how to learn a second language using what he knows in his first language. In order to achieve understanding, participants are using paraphrase, translation, repetition, different repair procedures, and clarification requests in both languages. Yves is also learning that code-switching is acceptable in this context for getting his thoughts across.

CONCLUSIONS

The importance of input in terms of understanding the verbal routines that take place in multilingual households cannot be underestimated (Genesee, 1989; Goodz, 1989; Kulick, 1992), and we can see from these few examples that changes in setting, topic, and participants are not the only reasons for code-switching. In these exchanges learning another language and communicating one's thoughts are good reasons to shift from one code to another. This suggests that we must broaden our notion of context, although for many it is already too slippery and all-inclusive. But what I am referring to specifically are three particular aspects of context.

First, we need to broaden our notion of the unit of analysis to include spontaneous conversations analyzed in terms of the discourse sequencing. Second, we need to broaden our notions of relevant participants and include more of the voices that make up the verbal environment of the child. Not only in multilingual households but in monolingual households we need to acknowledge the multilingual, or multidialectal, input from the verbal environment and take into account the many nonstandard English speakers and non-English speakers who are employed to take care of the children. We cannot ignore the fact that these caregivers speak to other people's children similarly to the ways in which they speak to their own, using the language(s) in which they are most comfortable and that they feel to be the most appropriate to express what they need to say. These languages, like these other caregivers themselves, have been kept hidden in the psycholinguistic and sociolinguistic literature. But they need not be. Third, we must directly investigate their speech practices beyond self-reported speech preferences and use. Language socialization, an approach that focuses on the verbal environment of the young child and is based on ethnographic methods, seems to be the best perspective for such an enterprise. We just might find that language learning situations for many monolingual children are much more bi- and multilingual (and multicultural) than we have previously thought. Although this makes for more complex methods and messier theories, we might just find some of the missing pieces that help complete the sociolinguistic and psycholinguistic puzzles that we have been constructing for years.

NOTES

I would like to thank the many Haitians who assisted in this research project by letting me visit their homes and record their everyday activities. Their names have been changed to protect their privacy. Special thanks go to Rachelle Doucet and Edwidge Bryant who helped me understand Kreyòl, among other things. I would also like to thank the Spencer Foundation and New York University's Research Challenge Fund for providing funding for this project on language socialization in Kreyòl-speaking families. An earlier version of this paper was presented at the New York Child Language meeting February 1991. My thanks to Patsy Lightbown for helpful suggestions early on, to Lois Bloom for her continued support, and to Elinor Ochs and the editors of this volume for comments that improved the clarity of my thoughts.

 1.   These were longitudinal case studies, often carried out by a parent-researcher, documenting the acquisition of two languages. See de Houwer (1990, Chapter 2) and Romaine (1989, Chapter 5) for discussions of methodological and theoretical aspects of these studies.

 2.   For research done in the United States, Amastae and Elías-Olivares, 1983; Duran, 1981; Elías-Olivares, 1983; and Zentella, 1981, 1990, are excellent sources.

 3.   Relatively low mixing rates are also reported by Bergman, 1976; Garcia, 1980; Lindholm, 1980; Lindholm and Padilla, 1978; and Padilla and Liebman, 1975.

 4.   Transcription conventions: Unintelligible utterances are indicated by—/. Most exchanges in these examples are between Yves and his aunt; / between words indicates a self-repair. The word 'okay' is widely used by Haitians living in New York in ways similar to that of native English speakers and thus is not counted as a code-switch in this speech community.

REFERENCES

Amastae, J., & Elías-Olivares, L. (Eds.). (1983). *Sociolinguistic aspects of Spanish in the United States.* New York: Cambridge University Press.

Auer, J. C. P. (1988). A conversational analytic approach to code-switching and transfer. In M. Heller (Ed.), *Codeswitching: Anthropological and sociolinguistic perspectives* (pp. 187–213). Berlin: Mouton.

Bateson, G. (1972). *Steps to an ecology of mind.* New York: Ballantine Books.

Bergman, C. (1976). Interference vs. independent development in infant bilingualism. In G. Keller (Ed.) *Bilingualism in the bicentenial and beyond* (pp. 87–96). New York: Bilingual Press.

Blom, J. P., & Gumperz, J. (1972). Social meaning in linguistic structures: Code-switching in Norway. In J. Gumperz & D. Hymes (Eds.), *Directions in sociolinguistics.* New York: Holt, Rinehart and Winston.

Boggs, S. (1985). *Speaking, relating, and learning: A study of Hawaiian children at home and at school.* Norwood, NJ: Ablex.

Cherry, L. (1979). The role of adults' requests for clarification in the language development of children. In R. Freedle (Ed.), *New directions in discourse processes* (Vol. 2). Norwood, NJ: Ablex.

Clancy, P. (1986). The acquisition of communicative style in Japanese. In B. B. Schieffelin & E. Ochs (Eds.), *Language socialization across cultures.* New York: Cambridge University Press.

Crago, M. (1988). *Cultural context in communicative interaction of Inuit children.* Ph.D. dissertation. McGill University.

de Houwer, A. (1990). *The acquisition of two languages from birth: A case study.* New York: Cambridge University Press.

Diaz, R. (1985). The intellectual power of bilingualism. *The Quarterly Newsletter of the Laboratory of Comparative Human Cognition,* (1), 16–22.

Doyle, A., Champagne, M., & Segalowitz, N. (1978). Some issues in the assessment of linguistic consequences of early bilingualism. In M. Paradis (Ed.), *Aspects of bilingualism* (pp. 13–20). Columbia, SC: Hornbeam Press.

Duran, R. (Ed.). (1981). *Latino language and communicative behavior.* Norwood, NJ: Ablex.

Elías-Olivares, L. (Ed.). (1983). *Spanish in the U.S. setting: Beyond the southwest.* Riverside, CA: National Clearinghouse for Bilingual Education.

Erin-Tripp, S. (1981). Social process in first- and second-language learning. In H. Winitz (Ed.), *Native language and foreign language acquisition* (Vol. 379, pp. 33–47). New York: Annals of the New York Academy of Sciences.

Fillmore, L. (1976). *The second time around: Cognitive and social strategies in second language acquisition.* Ph.D. dissertation, Stanford University.

Gal, S. (1987). Codeswitching and consciousness in the European periphery. *American Ethnologist, 14* (4), 637–653.

Garcia, E. (1980). The functions of language switching during bilingual mother–child interactions. *Journal of Multilingual and Multicultural Development, 1* (3), 243–252.

Garvey, C. (1977). The contingent query: A dependent act in conversation. In M. Lewis & L. Rosenblum (Eds.), *Interaction, conversation and the development of language.* New York: Wiley.

Genesee, F. (1989). Early bilingual development: One language or two? *Journal of Child Language, 16,* 161–179.

Genishi, C. (1981). Code-switching in Chicano six-year olds. In R. Duran (Ed.), *Latino language and communicative behavior* (pp. 133–152). Norwood, NJ: Ablex.

Golinkoff, R. (1983). The preverbal negotiation of failed messages. In R. Golinkoff (Ed.), *The transition from prelinguistic to linguistic communication* (pp. 57–78). Hillsdale, NJ: Lawrence Erlbaum.

Goodwin, C., & Heritage, J. (1990). Conversation analysis. In B. Siegel (Ed.), *Annual review of anthropology.* Palo Alto, CA: Annual Reviews.

Goodz, N. (1989). Parental language mixing in bilingual families. *Infant Mental Health Journal, 10* (1), 25–44.

Grosjean, F. (1982). *Life with two languages.* Cambridge, MA: Harvard University Press.

Gumperz, J. (1967). Linguistic markers of bilingual communication. *Journal of Social Issues, 23,* 137–153.

Gumperz, J. (1982). *Discourse strategies.* New York: Cambridge University Press.

Gumperz, J., & Hymes, D. (Eds.). (1972). *Directions in sociolinguistics.* New York: Holt, Rinehart and Winston.

Hakuta, K. (1986). *The mirror for language: The debate on bilingualism.* New York: Basic Books.

Hamers, J., & Blanc, M. (1989). *Bilinguality and bilingualism.* New York: Cambridge University Press.

Heath, S. (1983). *Ways with words: Language, life and work in communities and classrooms*. New York: Cambridge University Press.

Heller, M. (Ed.). (1988). *Codeswitching: Anthropological and sociolinguistic perspectives*. Berlin: Mouton.

Huertas-Macias, (1981). Code-switching: All in the family. In R. Duran (Ed.), *Latino language and communicative behavior* (pp. 153–168). Norwood, NJ: Ablex.

Hyltenstam, K., & Obler, L. (Eds.). (1989). *Bilingualism across the lifespan: Aspects of acquisition, maturity and loss*. New York: Cambridge University Press.

Keller, G., Teschner, R., & Viera, S. (Eds.). (1976). *Bilingualism in the bicentenial and beyond*. Jamaica, NY: Bilingual Press.

Kulick, D. (1992). *Language shift and cultural reproduction: Socialization, self and syncretism in a Papua New Guinean village*. New York: Cambridge University Press.

Leopold, W. F. (1939–1949). *Speech development in a bilingual child* (4 vols.). Evanston, IL: Northwestern University Press.

Lindholm, K. (1980). Bilingual children: Some interpretations of cognitive development. In K. E. Nelson (Ed.), *Children's language*. (Vol. 2, pp. 215–266). New York: Gardner Press.

Lindholm, K., & Padilla, A. (1978). Language mixing in bilingual children. *Journal of Child Language, 5*, 327–335.

McClure, E. (1977). Aspects of code-switching in the discourse of bilingual Mexican-American children. In M. Saville-Troike (Ed.), *Linguistics and anthropology* (pp. 93–115). Washington, D.C.: Georgetown University Round Table on Languages and Linguistics.

McClure, E. (1981). Formal and functional aspects of code-switched discourse of bilingual children. In R. Duran (Ed.), *Latino language and communicative behavior* (pp. 69–94). Norwood, NJ: Ablex.

McLaughlin, B. (1981). Differences and similarities between first- and second-language learning. In H. Winitz (Ed.), *Native language and foreign language acquisition* (Vol. 379, pp. 23–32). New York: Annals of the New York Academy of Sciences.

McLaughlin, B. (1984). Early bilingualism: Methodological and theoretical issues. In M. Paradis & Y. Lebrun (Eds.), *Early bilingualism and child development* (pp. 19–45). Lisse: Swets & Zeitlinger.

Miller, P. (1982). *Amy, Wendy and Beth: Language learning in South Baltimore*. Austin: University of Texas Press.

Miller, P., Potts, R., Fung, H., Hoogstra, E., & Mintz, J. (1990). Narrative practices and the social construction of self in childhood. *American Ethnologist, 17* (2), 292–311.

Ochs, E. (1988). *Culture and language development*. New York: Cambridge University Press.

Ochs, E. (1990). Misunderstanding children. In N. Coupland, H. Giles, & J. Wieman (Eds.), *Handbook of miscommunication*. Clevedon, UK: Multilingual Matters, Ltd.

Ochs, E., & Schieffelin, B. B. (1984). Language acquisition and socialization: Three developmental stories and their implications. In R. Shweder & R. LeVine (eds.), *Culture theory: Essays on mind, self and emotion* (pp. 276–320). New York: Cambridge University Press.

Padilla, A. M., & Liebman, E. (1975). Language acquisition in the bilingual child. *Bilingual Review, 2* (1–2), 34–55.

Padilla, A. M., & Lindholm, E. (1976). Acquisition of bilingualism: A descriptive analysis of the linguistic structures of Spanish/English speaking children. In G. Keller, R. Teschner, & S. Viera (Eds.), *Bilingualism in the bicentenial and beyond.* Jamaica, NY: Bilingual Press.

Poplack, S. (1981). Syntactic structure and social function of code-switching. In R. Duran (Ed.), *Latino language and communicative behavior* (pp. 169–184). Norwood, NJ: Ablex.

Redlinger, W., & Park, T-Z. (1980). Language mixing in young bilinguals. *Journal of Child Language, 7,* 337–352.

Rogoff, B. (1989). *Apprenticeship in thinking.* Oxford: Oxford University Press.

Romaine, S. (1989). *Bilingualism.* Oxford: Basil Blackwell.

Ronjat, J. (1913). *Le développment du langage observé chez un enfant bilingue.* Paris: Champion.

Schegloff, E., Jefferson, G., & Sacks, H. (1977). The preference for self-correction in the organization of repair in conversation. *Language, 53,* 361–382.

Schieffelin, B. B. (1990). *The give and take of everyday life: Language socialization of Kaluli children.* New York: Cambridge University Press.

Schieffelin, B. B. (in prep.) Language socialization in more than one language. In D. Slobin et al. (Eds.), *Festschrift in honor of Susan Ervin-Tripp.*

Schieffelin, B. B., & Ochs, E. (Eds.). (1986a). *Language socialization across cultures.* New York: Cambridge University Press.

Schieffelin, B. B., & Ochs, E. (1986b). Language socialization. In B. Siegel (Ed.), *Annual review of anthropology,* (pp. 163–191). Palo Alto, CA: Annual Reviews.

Snow, C. (1977). The development of conversations between mothers and babies. *Journal of Child Language, 4,* 1–22.

Snow, C., & Ferguson, C. (Eds.) (1977). *Talking to children: Language input and acquisition.* New York: Cambridge University Press.

Volterra, V., & Taeschner, T. (1978). The acquisition and development of language in bilingual children. *Journal of Child Language, 5,* 311–326.

Watson-Gegeo, K., & Gegeo, D. (1986). Calling out and repeating routines of Kwara'ae children's language socialization. In B. B. Schieffelin & E. Ochs (Eds.). *Language socialization across cultures.* New York: Cambridge University Press.

Weinreich, U. (1953). *Languages in contact.* The Hague: Mouton.

Zentella, A. C. (1981). *"Hablamos los dos. We speak both": Growing up bilingual in el Barrio.* Ph.D. dissertation, University of Pennsylvania.

Zentella, A. C. (1990). Integrating qualitative and quantitative methods in the study of bilingual code-switching. In E. Bendix (Ed.). *The uses of linguistics.* (Vol. 583, pp. 75–92). New York: Annals of the New York Academy of Sciences.

chapter 4

CULTURE, CONVERSATION, AND INTERACTION

Implications for Intervention

Martha B. Crago and Alice Eriks-Brophy

INTRODUCTION

It is now an apt time to write about the culture of conversations with Native American children. It was 500 years ago that white men had their first conversations with Native Americans and Native Canadians. In a recent survey (Warren 1990) asked Native Americans the following question: "In what way would you characterize the Quincentenary?" Seventy percent of the respondents selected the description of either "500 years of native people's resistance to colonization" or "an anniversary of a holocaust." Only 20 percent picked "a commemoration of a cultural encounter," and only 6 percent considered it a "celebration of discovery." If Native people think of their encounters with the dominant American and Canadian society as genocidal and colonialistic, then it is important to inspect the nature of the conversations that comprise these encounters.

This chapter, then, has to do with how cultural differences, unintentional cultural misunderstandings, and cultural dominance can be played out in the conversations of clinical and educational encounters. It is also, and just as much, about how meaningful and culturally sensitive conversations can be co-constructed and used in education and intervention with children and their families.

THEORETICAL APPROACHES TO CULTURE
AND CONVERSATIONS WITH CHILDREN

It has been recognized for some time by sociolinguists and ethnographers of speaking that conversations are culturally variable events (Gumperz, 1982; Hymes, 1974). People's strategies for discourse show that there is an enormous range of signalling devices available within a culture and a wide variation in rules for speaking across cultures. Furthermore, these devices and rules are related to cultural values and social norms, as well as to the status and roles of the conversationalists. They thereby influence who can speak to whom, about what, and in what way.

The nature of conversations with children has also been documented to be a culturally variable phenomenon (Crago, 1988, 1992; Heath, 1983; Ochs, 1988; Schieffelin, 1990), one in which the values of a culture influence the communicative interactions that caregivers have with their children. Children are socialized into their culture by the ways in which their caregivers and peers talk to them and guide them to participate in conversations. Who guides the child, to what ends, and in what ways varies across cultures (Rogoff, 1990). Implicit in early conversations with children is the creation of specific cultural membership.

The socialization of children extends beyond the family. It includes the social and cultural world of the school and, for communicatively impaired children, it includes the world of clinical intervention. Literature on classroom practice has pointed out how certain cultural differences between a teacher and the students can lead to unsuccessful educational outcomes (Cazden, 1988; Erickson, 1987; Philips, 1983). Differences between children's and teachers' ideas of communicative interaction and differences in their expected patterns of discourse lead to deficit interpretations by teachers. The conversations of classrooms, then, can be considered a secondary form of socialization for certain children. For these children, the ability to engage in such conversations in expected ways and to learn through them is not a straightforward process. It can involve the risk of cultural loss and it certainly involves an extra load of learning. Another very real risk is that cultural differences can become boundaries between the teachers and the students with ensuing resistance to schooling on the part of the learners or a pressure for assimilation imposed by teachers upon the children and their families. Cazden (1988) in her book on classroom discourse calls for a reconceptualization or recontextualization of the ways of interacting with children from various cultures in the classroom. This implies that teachers should transform classroom practices to be congruent with children's ways of talking.

There is another set of pertinent theories that describes cultural differences in conversations in terms of dominance and power. Bourdieu and Passeron (1990) have articulated a theory that interprets educational institutions as an extension of the dominant culture. The dominant culture is seen as imposing its norms and ways of interacting (including conversing) upon non-dominant members of the society. Through schooling, members of the dominant culture reproduce and ensure their hold on their position of dominance. Lack of conformity to the linguistic and interactional patterns of what these writers call the "educational authority" can lead to lack of success in school and a future lack of success in the marketplace. Gal (1989) has referred to a phenomenon that she calls "cultural capital." Cultural capital includes the ability to converse in ways that conform with the dominant culture. It is, in a sense, the wherewithal to succeed in school and the marketplace. Certain nonmainstream members of the North American society do not possess the same cultural capital that members of the dominant society possess.

This chapter describes some properties of the home and school conversations of aboriginal members of Canadian society from the perspective of cultural differences and issues of social dominance. In doing so, the chapter represents an example of how information on the cultural dimensions of communication can be gathered using ethnographic methodology. Such information derived from the Inuit people has been necessary in order to transform the communicative interaction of clinical and educational practice in culturally appropriate and meaningful ways. Clinicians working with other nondominant cultural groups need to gather similar information in order to transform their own clinical practice. The detail associated with each cultural group will vary. This chapter describes some kinds of communicative interactions that are important in the Inuit culture, interactions that reveal central issues for intervention and classroom practice.

CULTURAL VARIATION IN INTERACTION: AN INUIT EXAMPLE

The interactions reported in this chapter took place in two communities of Northern Quebec: Kangirsuk and Quaqtaq. These are small Inuit communities (population 325 and 200, respectively) in which the native language, Inuktitut, is spoken on a routine basis. Inuit people are frequently called Eskimos by mainstream North Americans. However, the word *eskimo*, meaning "raw meat eaters," comes from the Cree language and it is not used by Inuit to refer to themselves. Instead they use the word *Inuit* (*Inuk* in the singular), which, in their language, means "the people."

Formal schooling came to this region in the mid-1960s, forcing the population to abandon its nomadic way of life and leading to the inception of communities with permanent houses. The Inuit in Northern Quebec now run their own schools in which kindergarten through Grade 2 are taught in Inuktitut by Inuit teachers who have received their teacher education in Inuktitut through courses given in Northern Quebec under the aegis of McGill University.

Home Interactions

This first set of interactions was collected in the homes of four children between the ages of one and two. They are excerpts from 80 hours of video-tapes made over a year's time. Two of the mothers in the study had, according to Inuit custom, adopted their children (Crago, 1988); these women were in their late forties. The other two mothers were in their early twenties. Three of the mothers lived in extended family groupings and the other one lived with her husband and small daughter. Such a nuclear family unit was still a rarity in Northern Quebec in 1986 when this study took place.

Nonverbal modelling. Demonstrations done by a competent cultural member or modelling has been a major style of learning and teaching in Inuit homes. The word *imaak* ("like that") is frequently used with children when instructing them in a task. The following episode lasted for no more than 10 minutes and was accompanied by this kind of teaching–learning conversation. Although it is atypical in that it involved toy play, it illustrates the use of nonverbal modelling.

Suusi: 1.3 years

[Suusi and her mother are sitting on the floor. The mother takes a stacking toy and shows the child how it goes together.]

Mo: Takugunai.   (Look)
       Imaak.   (Like this)
       Una, hai.   (This one, hey)
       Atii.   (Come on)
       Atii.   (Come on)

What makes this type of modelling interaction different from Anglo teaching styles is its succinctness and focus on nonverbal demonstration rather than verbal explanation.

Repetition routines with siblings. Young Inuit children are also en-couraged to model verbal behavior on that of their older siblings through repetition or imitation routines. In these routines, the children are instructed to say something by being told to repeat after their caregivers. For verbal material, Inuit instruct their children to model or repeat by saying *lalaurit* ("say it like this"). Verbal repetition routines used with the four Inuit children we studied were primarily used by young mothers, teen-aged caregivers, or siblings. They were of two main types: routines that often took place in triadic settings in which the child was instructed on how to greet and acknowledge greetings, and repetition routines used to get young children to say phrases in English, including politeness conventions and counting.

Learning to greet, by adding the ending -ai to a name or kinship term and to acknowledge greetings with the word ah, is one of the verbal concomitants to learning to take one's place in the community and family. Inuit kinship terms differ depending on both the sex of the speaker and of the addressee. From both this example and the next one, it is evident that repetition routines function as a kind of miniscript (Peters & Boggs, 1986) for learning greetings. These greeting routines help to situate young Inuit children socially by leading to the acquisition, at two years of age, of several kin terms, the properties of deixis, turn taking, and the importance of acknowledgment. No other single language feature was so extensively structured for the children. The following conversational exchange had a total of 27 interchanges, only a few of which are shown here.

[Suusi and her mother have been eating lunch at Suusi's grandmother's house. Two of her cousins, Natali (4 years old) and Gabriel (3 years old), come in and join them. The children are all sitting at the table.]

Mo:	Qatailalauruk.	(Say, 'greetings girl cousin')
Su:	Huh?	
Mo:	Qatailalauruk.	(Say, 'greetings girl cousin')
	Inna.	(That one)
	Qatailalauruk.	(Say to her, 'greetings girl cousin')
	Qatailalauruk.	(Say to her, 'greetings girl cousin')
Su:	Qatai.	(Greetings girl cousin)
Mo to Natali:		
	Anngaguk.	(Reply to her)
	Aahlalaurit.	(Say, 'aah to her')
Su:	Aah.	[acknowledgment]
Mo:	Qataapiaialalauruk.	(Say to her, 'greetings pretty girl cousin')
	Inna.	(Go on)
Su:	Qatai.	(Greetings girl cousin)
Mo:	Natalii angirruk.	(Natalii, reply to her)
	Qatapiailagu, Natalii.	(Natalii, say, 'pretty girl cousin')

The next example of a child's being instructed to greet and to acknowledge the greeting demonstrates the deictic properties that are taught in such imitative routines.

Jini: 1.8 years [Jini hands her older sister, Miaji, a banana. Miaji pretends the banana is a telephone and talks into it.]

Mi:		Jiniai.	(Greetings Jini)
Ji:		Aah.	[acknowledgment]
Mi:		Ailalaurit.	(Say, 'greetings')
Ji:		Ai.	(Greetings)
Mi:		Aah. Jiniai.	([Acknowledgment]. Greetings Jini)
Ji:	*	Jiniai.	(Greetings Jini)
Mi:	*	Aah. Miajiai.	(Greetings Miaji)

Ji: Miaji.   (Miaji)
Mi: Aah.   [acknowledgment]

What begins as a repetition routine breaks down if the child can only repeat
and cannot understand how what he or she has to say differs from what the
other person has to say. Jini has not yet acquired the deictic understanding
necessary to maintain the routine as a successful two-party exchange (* =
the inappropriate utterances). The older sister turns Jini's error into a tease
or joke. In the end, Jini finally converts the situation into an appropriate two-
party format. It is interesting to note that Jini did not express deixis with
personal pronoun affixes at this age. Three months later, when she was capable
of handling the deictic properties of greeting routines, Jini still did not use
personal pronoun affixes. Jini's mother did not engage in any greeting routines
with her daughter. This seemed to be the domain of the sibling caregiver
rather than that of an older mother.

Hierarchies of communicative partners.   Inuit traditionally lived in extended multiage family groupings. Many still do. Such families have a wide
variety of communicative interaction in them. What is intriguing is who talks
and who listens and with whom. Who are the spectators and who are the
performers and in whose company? Such families are a rich environment for
children to learn by watching and listening to the interactions of others. There
are family members with varying degrees of competence and status to relate
to and to watch as they relate to each other.

In general, children talk to children. Older siblings have communicative
interactions with young children that include teasing and repetition routines.
Adults talk with adults, sometimes at length and sometimes with great economy of speech. Adults have communicative interactions with young children
that include directives, affectionate talk, teasing, ignoring their children's
intrusions and questions, and companionable and disciplinary silence. Children talk with adults but not usually by asking questions nor when adults are
conversing. In most homes children are omnipresent. By a process of exclusion, they are kept from hearing what is too adult for their ears and socialized
to the idea that older people are shown respect for their knowledge by their
roles of performer and talker. In the daily running of the home, there is a
sort of hierarchy of child care whereby an older person will relate less directly
to a young child if a sibling caregiver is present. When the sibling caregiver
is present, the adult can retire.

One older mother expressed the differences in roles of conversational
partners with Inuit children in the following way:

Qaajia: If the child has siblings she is taught more to talk by them; when they look
after their younger siblings they talk to them. The mother talks less to the baby than
the one who is taking care of the baby for her. The mother teaches the child to talk
less than the person who is looking after the baby.

Interviewer: Is it the same as the mother, the way the sibling teaches the child to talk?

Qaajia: The older sibling teaches the younger sibling in different ways. The mother talks about the more important things to the child.

Interviewer: What are the more important things?

Qaajia: These different things we have to work on, like obeying, helping others. Obeying what you are told to do is heavier when it is your mother telling you.

The small nuclear family is a very recent but growing phenomenon in Northern Quebec. Some young couples and even single mothers are eager to have their own houses or apartments. More and more of these housing units are being built for them. As this happens, the children have less and less of the rich tapestry of relationships and communicative interactions in their own home to watch, listen to, engage in, and learn from. The conversational patterns are likely to change accordingly, requiring yet another transformation in school to provide cultural congruence.

Interaction in silence. Older mothers often interacted with their children in silence. The following episode is typical of interaction between children and their older mothers.

Jini: 1.3 years [Jini and her mother are sitting in a bedroom watching TV. The child gets up and toddles out into the living room. She fusses. Qaajia gets up and slowly follows the child, saying nothing. They continue through the living room to the kitchen. Qaajia begins to prepare a bottle of diluted canned milk for Jini. Jini spots an open door to the cupboard under the sink. She goes in with the bottles of detergent and other cleaning products. Her mother looks at her and smiles at her through the half-shut cupboard door.]

Mother: Bye.

[The mother continues preparing the milk in silence, keeping an eye on the cupboard door. When the bottle is ready, she holds it up in front of the cupboard door so that the child can see it. The child emerges, takes the bottle, begins drinking, and turns around to open the cupboard door. Her mother has closed it. The child takes one handle and pulls. The mother's knee blocks the door from opening. The child pulls again. The mother's thumb blocks the door. The mother's other arm gently turns the child toward the living room.]

The contrast between one of the authors' (MBC) reactions in a situation of conflict with her three-year-old son and Qaajia's reaction to her two-year-old daughter is demonstrated in this next interchange:

[I took Peter with me to Qaajia's house this afternoon. Qaajia was sitting and sewing in the living room. Peter and Jini (2,0 years old) decided that they wanted to play with the same ball, but not together. Peter took it and Jini screamed.]

MBC: Peter, play with Jini. Throw her the ball.

[Peter threw the ball to Jini. Jini grabbed it and ran away. Qaajia was silent. Peter ran after her and grabbed the ball. Jini screamed. Peter screamed. Qaajia called the community radio to announce that Miaji, her teen-aged daughter should come home.]

MBC: Peter you have to share with Jini. If you can't share you'll have to go back to Betsy's house. Why don't you play with Jini? Don't grab the ball.

[The two children continued to tussle over the ball. Qaajia went on sewing. Miaji walked in. Qaajia asked her to find the second identical ball that they had. Miaji did. Qaajia gave it to Jini. Jini threw it aside and went to grab Peter's ball. Peter screamed and pinched her.]

MBC: Peter, for heaven's sake. Why don't you take the other ball? It's just the same. Really, if you can't stop this nonsense, I'm going to take you to Betsy's. Remember, I said you could come with me, if you behaved yourself.

[Qaajia continued sewing. Jini wailed and flung herself on the sofa: She screamed:]

Ji: Anaana (Mother) . . .

[Qaajia went on sewing. Jini walked toward the bedroom crying, went and lay on the bed. Qaajia brought her a bottle of milk, gave it to her in silence, and walked out. Jini drank the bottle and fell asleep. I took Peter by the hand and went to Betsy's, lecturing him the whole way there.]

An Inuk colleague interpreted this contrast in style in the following way:

That is how our parents show us who is boss . . . with their silence.

This episode also indicated how one Inuk parent guided her child toward cooperative, sharing behavior by negatively sanctioning selfish behavior. Sharing is a fundamental value in Inuit society as is cooperative group activity.

School Conversations

Interactions in the classrooms of Inuit teachers mirror some of the properties of communicative interaction in traditional Inuit homes. The following excerpts are taken from over 50 hours of videotaping and several hundred hours of observation of five Inuit teachers who taught the four children documented in the home study.

A sample classroom interaction. These first teaching–learning conversations come from the classroom of an older woman. In her Grade 1–2 class, the teacher and her students spent much time in joint attention to an object or activity, seldom gazing directly at each other. For example, when the teacher was involved in making paper flowers out of egg cartons, the students observed the varieties of flowers that the teacher constructed and, then, copied them. The teacher rarely looked up at the students and indeed rarely spoke. At one point, when the teacher had made a particularly beautiful flower, she held it up to the group and drew in her breath loudly while looking at the flower. The students looked at the flower and many of them then attempted to copy the teacher's idea. Most of this activity took place in silence, with attention focused almost exclusively on the objects and materials. At the conclusion of the lesson, the teacher directed one student to get a large can from the bookcase. All the egg carton flowers were placed together in this can. There was no attempt to identify any single flower as belonging to any one student. No one asked to keep a flower or to place any one of them in an individual container.

The egg carton flower lesson exemplifies how traditional Inuit values and cultural ways can be incorporated into classroom interactions, including the notions of learning by looking, teaching through modelling and not through talk, and the respectful silence of children in the presence of an elder. In addition, this classroom lesson includes the notions of cooperation and lack of emphasis on possession and individuality, values that are similar to those that parents emphasize in the home.

Teacher use of peer models.   During interviews conducted with the Inuit teachers, they described one of their most important roles in the classroom to be the facilitation of peer exchanges and not primarily teacher control or strict transmission of knowledge.

Students were frequently encouraged to listen to their peers and were rarely scolded or corrected by the teacher. Instead, they were quietly and often subtly guided to peer models who were completing the activity as desired or who had the correct response. In addition to the positive models provided by the peer group, several of the more experienced teachers stressed the responsibility of the group in peer tutoring as well as the importance of peer cooperation, membership, and encouragement. Peer talk and peer interactions were consciously promoted and highly valued in all the Inuit classrooms we studied. As one teacher commented:

> Students can't learn by themselves. No one pushes them to learn if they are by themselves, listening only to the teacher and not to each other. Students don't learn alone. They need the others to learn from.

During a visit to a Montreal-based classroom, one of the Inuit teachers who was very involved in the research commented that she felt the Montreal teacher corrected the children's reading errors unnecessarily. In her own classroom, she said, she encouraged her students to correct each other's reading errors, and in fact she did not feel that this way of correcting errors was an appropriate role for the teacher, as it did not encourage the children to listen to and help each other. This teacher would intentionally make errors in her use of vocabulary or mention facts that were incorrect in her teaching. The students would then correct her by calling out the proper answer or fact. When asked why she did this, she replied that rather than the teacher holding sole responsibility for correcting the group, she wanted to encourage the students to listen to others and to feel free to correct each other's errors. She felt that this way of teaching encouraged students to take a more active and responsible role in the learning for themselves and also for all the members of the group.

Another means Inuit teachers used to promote equality and cooperation among group members was through use of what Mehan (1979) has called the "invitation to reply" rather than the "invitation to bid" format of elicitation, as well as through avoidance of overt praise or evaluation for individual group members. The six Inuit teachers involved in our study typically directed questions to the group as a whole and only rarely singled out students to respond individually to teacher-initiated questions. Although teachers initiated the topic of a lesson, they never attempted to control students' contributions by requiring bids for turns through the raising of hands in the "invitation to bid" format. The focus in classroom interaction was on the peer group and not on individual group members. This was accomplished through use of a variation of Mehan's (1979) Initiation–Response–Evaluation (IRE) sequences that Eriks-Brophy (1992) has called "Inuit IR routines." In these IR routines, the teacher initiated a sequence and the students called out the answer as a group. The teacher did not select an individual speaker and made no overt evaluation of the correctness of the group reply after an elicitation.

Inuit teachers did not require strict adherence to topic in class discussions. Student contributions to a lesson topic were easily accepted, incorporated, and expanded upon by the teachers.

Kindergarten: Oral lesson on animals

Teacher: Do Inuit people eat wolves?

Students: No.

Teacher: What do they do with them?

Students: Fur.

Student: Wolves are grey.

Teacher: Yes, they are grey. The wolves are grey, right?

Students: Yes.

Student: And they are white, too.

Students: White.

Student: And black.

Teacher: Yes.

Student: Some are brown, too.

Student: My father got a big one.

Teacher: Oh, yes?

Student: Harry got one, too.

The teaching–learning conversations of Inuit teachers, then, differed in a number of ways from those described by Mehan (1979) for mainstream teachers. Seeing how typical classroom conversations have been transformed or reconceptualized by these native teachers helps reveal that "the classroom environment is not simply a given, external object, but a socially generated pattern in whose maintenance and construction students (and teachers) play a part" (Bredo, Henry, & McDermott, 1991, p. 324).

Examination and delineation of a set of cultural practices can serve not only to make communicative practices explicit, both for the members of the culture and for others, but they can also be used as a means to strengthen them. Documenting family and classroom discourse and interactional patterns in diverse cultural groups will not only promote harmony between the home and classroom, but also promote and maintain the status of culturally specific patterns of conversation.

THE CULTURAL TRANSFORMATION OF CLINICAL CONVERSATIONS

How then can the conversations and interactions of clinical intervention be reconceptualized or recontextualized? How can patterns of interaction and forms of conversation be generated that will most appropriately serve the intervention needs, the cultural needs, and the social needs of our clients?

It is inappropriate to regard speech-language pathologists (SLPs) as solely responsible for the creation of culturally adapted programs (Crago & Cole, 1991). Most clinicians are from the mainstream culture and they know best how to create intervention programs that are suited to their own cultural backgrounds. There are far too few SLPs who come from outside the mainstream. One alternative to this impasse is to work collaboratively with families and other culture members to co-construct intervention that is appropriate for their children. If an interactional framework for intervention in which naturalistic ways of conversing is the objective, information is needed about natural conversational formats, usual situations, and typical conversational partners for the children being served (see Crago & Cole, 1991, for a questionnaire to elicit this information).

One way to reconceptualize clinical practice is to consider the implications of a sociocultural approach to clinical practice (see Table 4–1). Snow,
Midkiff-Borunda, Small, and Proctor (1984) have described behavioral, psycholinguistic, and sociolinguistic approaches to language intervention with
children. Their work does not consider the role of cultural context for intervention. The clinical philosophies and clinical examples that they cite are
congruent with and reflect the North American white middle-class culture.
In this sense, their work might be said to be highly culturally contextualized,
but contextualized in only one culture. It is interesting to reframe some of
Snow et al.'s categories keeping cultural issues in mind and seeing how their
categories work for a culture such as the Inuit one.

Clinicians working from such sociocultural framework would not, for
instance, specify particular activities and communicative partners, as Snow et
al. have done, since the appropriate methods would be highly variable across
cultures. In the Inuit culture, for example, sibling caregivers as well as children's peer groups might provide important interactants for intervention.
Reinforcement also needs to be seen as culturally variable. In the Inuit case,
it might consist of much less verbal evaluation on the part of a clinician and
of substituting peers to carry out modelling and corrections. The issue of who
does what that Snow et al. refer to as controlling the stimulus is also culturally
variable. In the Inuit culture, certain repetition routines are assigned to particular interactants, for example, to older siblings. These older siblings tend
to control the interactions of repetition routines by guiding and leading the
child through direct instruction of what to repeat. In such cases, the child's
lead is not followed in the same way that has been described for certain parent–
child intervention programs (Manolson, 1983). To the contrary, it is expected
that the children will model after more competent cultural members. In this
way, Inuit repetition routines introduce a new version of the imitation sequences that have previously been associated with the behavioral approach.

These repetition routines can also be referred to as "product oriented,"
to use Snow et al.'s term. In other words, a particular language outcome is
envisioned by the caregiver and children are prompted until they respond as
anticipated. This contrasts with the process orientation that Snow et al. described as characterizing the sociolinguistic approach. Process orientation
implies conversational exchanges between interlocutors in which no specific
outcome is envisioned by either partner. This kind of process orientation does
characterize some Inuit conversations, for instance, those that occur between
children and their peers. A sociocultural framework for interactions would,
then, encompass possibilities for both process and product orientations in
communicative exchanges.

Snow et al. (1984) showed how the sociolinguistic approach to intervention is structured around what they refer to as role exchange or the alternation of conversational roles between children and adults. In such role
exchanges, both partners are involved in expressive and receptive language

TABLE 4-1 Overview of Clinical Procedures

APPROACH	EXAMPLE	REFERENCE	CLINICAL PHILOSOPHY
Behavioral[a]	Stimulus—picture of boy with one foot in front of other Response—"the boy is walking" Reinforcement—gets a happy face Programmed instruction: Examples: Distar Fokes sentence builder Language Master	Skinner (1968)	Elicited imitation Drill with elaborate extrinsic reinforcement One communication partner Stimulus controlled by clinician Behaviorally based Product oriented Finite length of interaction
Psycholinguistic[a]	Stimulus—windup doll walking across table Response—"boy walking" Reinforcement—"Yeah, the boy is walking"	Bullowa (1979) McLean & Snyder-McLean (1978) Muma (1978) Muma, Pierce, & Muma (1983) Snow & Ferguson (1977) Wiig & Semel (1976, 1980)	Task at cognitive level of child Elicited imitation is meaning based Reinforcement is linguistic feedback—extensions and expansions of child's One or more communication partners Clinician/child in control of stimulus Meaning based Process/product oriented Finite or infintite length of interaction
Sociolinguistic[a]	Child—chooses windup toy to play with Clinician—holds windup doll ready to go Child—"walk doll" (duck, monkey, dog, etc.) Clinician—lets doll walk and says "the *doll* is *walking*" Child—"walk more" Clinician—acknowledges child's request for action by winding up doll again and expands utterance	Cook, Gumperz & Gumperz (1978) Craig (1983) Gallagher & Prutting (1983) McDermott, Gospodinoff, & Aron (1978) McDermott & Hood (1982) McLure & French (1981) Muma (1983) Shulz, Florio, & Erickson (1982) Waterson & Snow (1978) Wells (1981)	Task at cognitive and social level of the child Language models meaning based and functionally based Reinforcement is intrinsic to the conversation itself Stimulus chosen by child Turn taking in control of stimulus Socially based Process oriented Role exchange—receptive and expressive focus One or more communicative partners (to provide language models in conversational framework) Infinite length of interaction Interaction contingent on child's interests and negotiated meaning
Sociocultural	Culturally relevant activities and communicative partners	Cazden (1988) Crago (1992) Crago & Cole (1991) Erickson (1987) Eriks-Brophy (1992) Heath (1983) Hymes (1974) Ochs (1988) Philips (1983) Schieffelin (1990) Schieffelin & Ochs (1986) Taylor (1986)	Culturally appropriate task at child's social and cognitive level Language models meaning based, functionally based, and culturally based Reinforcement is intrinsic and culturally variable Stimuli control is culturally variable (e.g., can be peer negotiated or controlled by competent member) Turn taking is dependent on conversational partner Culturally and socially based Product or process oriented Role exchange is culturally variable—receptive and expressive focus depends on communicative partner, situation, and cultural values (e.g., not all interactions require role exchange or are realized through talk) One or more communicative partners (to provide culturally appropriate interactional hierarchy) Variable length of interaction Interaction contingent on the partner, the situation, and cultural values

[a]Taken from Snow et al. (1984)

behaviors. In Inuit society, however, certain conversational roles are situationally dependent and retained for adults only; for instance, entering into adult conversation is not an acceptable behavior for children. Other conversational roles alternate between Inuit children and adults. Furthermore, a variety of conversational partners are important in certain cultural groups, like the Inuit, in which an interactional hierarchy of communicating with children is more delineated than in the white middle-class culture. Snow et al. also refer to the length of the interaction. It, too, is culturally variable, depending on who the interactants are and on the situational context of the interaction. In the Inuit culture, certain interactions are negotiated in silence or are abbreviated by virtue of the interactant's being an older person. Others, between children and their peers, can be indefinite in length.

In summary, within a sociocultural framework, the nature of conversational interactions is contingent on the partner, the situation, and a particular group's cultural values surrounding the socialization of a child. These differences need to be reflected in clinical practice and in models for intervention. Our Inuit example has shown that categories associated with intervention in one culture do not necessarily work for another culture. The numerous dimensions of interaction—the linguistic, the social, the cognitive, **and the cultural**—all need to be integrated into both the theoretical approaches and the clinical philosophies of intervention with the communicatively disordered.

CONCLUSIONS

American and Canadian aboriginal groups differ considerably in the conversational and discourse practices used both in homes and in schools. This is due, in part, to cultural differences among the nations. It is also due to changes over time, to geographic location and relative remoteness from mainstream society, to the forces of assimilation and acculturation, as well as to certain native people's decisions to embrace modernism. The features of talk and silence described here are characteristic of some Inuit of Northern Quebec and may or may not apply to other groups or to all individuals within any particular group.

Cultural variability raises a number of considerations for clinicians serving populations with different cultural, conversational, and interactional exchanges. Can patterns of ignoring and obliterating differences be replaced by a celebration of variation? This chapter has shown that cultural variation can be incorporated into our classroom and clinical interactions. Classrooms and clinics need not be the metaphorical private dining clubs that Paley (Chapter 2) alluded to, in which Inuit come and are instructed to cook, set tables, and engage in mainstream conversations, while at home they have not traditionally cooked food nor sat at tables nor talked while they ate. However, if clinical and educational encounters are transformed into more relevant cultural events, are the children being placed on an ice flow unprepared to face the modern world, its schooling, and its economic realities? Can home cultural practices be developed as a strong base from which to encounter dominant societal practices? Is cultural duality in children a pipe dream? Is it even practical to conceive of language-impaired children learning two different sets of rules for constructing conversations?

We wish we had the answers to these questions.

REFERENCES

Bourdieu, P., & Passeron, J. C. (1990). *Reproduction in education, society, and culture.* Newbury Park, CA: Sage Publications.

Bredo, E., Henry, M., & McDermott, R. P. (1991). The cultural organization of teaching and learning. In M. Minami & B. P. Kennedy (Eds.), *Language issues in literary and bilingual multicultural education* (pp. 320–332). Cambridge, MA: Harvard University Press.

Cazden, C. (1988). *Classroom discourse.* Portsmouth, NH: Heinemann.

Crago, M. B. (1988). *Cultural context in communicative interaction of young Inuit children.* Unpublished doctoral dissertation, McGill University, Montreal.

Crago, M. B. (1992). Ethnography and language socialization: A cross-cultural perspective. *Topics in Language Disorders, 12* (3), 28–39.

Crago, M., & Cole, E. (1991). Using ethnography to bring children's communicative and cultural worlds into focus. In T. Gallagher (Ed.), *Pragmatics of language: Clinical practice issues* (pp. 99–132). San Diego, CA: Singular Publishing Group.

Erickson, F. (1987). Transformations and school success: The politics and culture of educational achievement. *Anthropology and Educational Quarterly, 18,* 335–357.

Eriks-Brophy, A. (1992). *The transformation of classroom discourse: An Inuit example.* Unpublished master's thesis, McGill University, Montreal.

Gal, S. (1989). Language and political economy. *Annual Review of Anthropology, 18,* 345–367.

Gumperz, J. J. (1982). *Discourse strategies.* New York: Cambridge University Press.

Heath, S. B. (1983). *Ways with words: Language, life and work in communities and classrooms.* New York: Cambridge University Press.

Hymes, D. H. (1974). The ethnography of speaking. In B. G. Blount (Ed.), *Language, culture, and society: A book of readings* (pp. 189–223). Cambridge, MA: Winthrop.

Manolson, A. (1983). *It takes two to talk: A Hanen early language parent guide book.* Toronto: Hanen Early Language Resource Center.

Mehan, H. (1979). *Learning lessons.* Cambridge, MA: Harvard University Press.

Ochs, E. (1988). *Culture and language development: Language acquisition and language socialization in a Samoan village.* New York: Cambridge University Press.

Peters, A., & Boggs, S. (1986). Interactional routines as cultural influences upon language acquisition. In B. B. Schieffelin & E. Ochs (Eds.). *Language socialization across cultures* (pp. 80–96). New York: Cambridge University Press.

Philips, S. U. (1983). *Invisible culture.* New York: Longman.

Rogoff, B. (1990). *Apprenticeship in thinking: Cognitive development in social context.* Oxford: Oxford University Press.

Schieffelin, B. (1990). *The give and take of everyday life.* New York: Cambridge University Press.

Schieffelin, B., & Ochs, E. (Eds.). (1986). *Language socialization across cultures.* New York: Cambridge University Press.

Snow, C., Midkiff-Borunda, S., Small, A., & Proctor, A. (1984). Therapy as social interaction: Analyzing the contexts for language remediation. *Topics in Language Disorders, 4* (3), 72–85.

Taylor, O. L. (1986). Issues, historical perspectives and conceptual framework. In O. L. Taylor (Ed.). *Treatment of communication disorders in culturally and linguistically diverse populations* (pp. 1–19). San Diego, CA: College-Hill Press.

Warren, D. (1990). American Indians and the Columbus quincentenary. *Northeast Indian Quarterly, 7* (3), 23–25.

chapter 5

WAYS TO TEACH CONVERSATION

Bonnie Brinton and Martin Fujiki

When the field of speech-language pathology was in its infancy, speech and language impairment was defined as some aspect of comprehension or production that compromised the interaction between speakers. For example, Van Riper (1939) noted that "Speech is defective when it deviates so far from the speech of other people in the group that it calls attention to itself, interferes with communication, or causes its possessor to be maladjusted to his environment" (p. 51).

Despite the reasonableness of this global view of communication disorders (Gallagher, 1991), much effort during the ensuing 30 years was devoted to separating and defining components and subcomponents of the communication process. Clinical intervention frequently involved the isolation, identification, and habilitation of individual behaviors that did not meet normative expectations. Within the bounds of this clinical philosophy, the actual use of targeted language behaviors to communicate was viewed as the final, and often untrained, step in the intervention process.

The last 15 years have witnessed a series of ideas and innovations in the treatment of language impairment labeled as "the pragmatics revolution" (Duchan, 1984). One of the major contributions of this revolution has been a reemphasis on the importance of communication in the context of social interaction. Researchers and clinicians have questioned the soundness of fragmented approaches and have focused attention on language in the actual settings in which it is used. From this perspective, assessment and intervention within the context of conversation have become increasingly important.

Although the consideration of communication in real conversations has great clinical potential, operationalizing this concept has not always been as straightforward as might be hoped. Many of the long-established protocols and clinical tools used in speech-language pathology cannot be effectively applied to the assessment and treatment of actual communication in conversation. A clinical approach committed to isolating, dividing, and conquering specific behaviors is not well equipped to capture the nature of the communicative process. Too frequently, "pragmatic" intervention has resulted in an attempt to compress conversation into a set of behaviors to be tested and taught, reinforced and shaped, perpetuated or extinguished.

Efforts to approach naturalistic interaction using traditional methods have been frustrated by the dynamic nature of communication. Resourceful clinical approaches are needed to meet the major challenges of (1) assessing communicative behaviors in a manner that maintains the integrity of the communication process and (2) facilitating, supporting, or compensating for impaired behaviors in a way that maximizes the ability of the individual to communicate.

In the face of these challenges, some scholars have abandoned the consideration of pragmatics or communication as an overriding construct, preferring to focus on the structural components of language. Others have adopted approaches so general that a child's strengths and weaknesses cannot be differentiated. We prefer a middle ground. We attempt to focus on and quantify specific behaviors. However, we work within the context of conversation. In all cases, the role played by specific behaviors in the communicative process is a primary concern.

We do not mean to imply that all children with language impairment have difficulty interacting in conversation, or that conversation should be the sole focus of intervention for all children. However, conversation is the best starting point from which to approach language impairment, regardless of whether the impairment involves structural or interactional components of language. We contend that it is possible to scrutinize aspects of language without isolating them and to evaluate the effects of certain behaviors on the interaction as a whole. Our ultimate objective is to facilitate the development of specific skills within conversational settings in a way that those skills will, in turn, enhance conversational interaction and communication. In this way, attention may be directed to a specific aspect of language without fragmenting the behavior from the whole.

The following sections provide a general overview of how assessment and intervention may be approached from this point of view. We then illustrate how these principles may be applied clinically by presenting a case study.

EVALUATION OF CONVERSATION

Traditionally, speech-language pathologists have relied heavily on standardized assessment instruments to diagnose communicative disorders. Although we often use these measures at some point in the evaluation process, formal tests do not constitute a viable starting point in the assessment of communicative behaviors. Rather, we begin by looking at the child's ability to take part in conversation. If a child has an impairment that interferes with communication, that deficit will most likely be manifest in conversational interaction.

The first step in assessing a child with suspected language impairment is to perform an initial screening. This screening consists of a number of questions focusing on the child's ability to interact in conversation. These questions are presented in Table 5–1.

Specific questions focus on the child's ability to share the talking time, to respond to feedback, to negotiate misunderstandings, and to cooperate with others in conversation. The questions are answered "yes" or "no" based on the clinician's observations and general impression of the child. Information gathered from parent and/or teacher report is also used in answering these questions.

If the information gathered from the screening suggests that further evaluation of conversation is warranted, the clinician may then examine specific behaviors in greater detail. The scope of this chapter does not allow elaboration on specific assessment procedures for conversational behaviors. However, there are a number of sources describing such methods, and the reader may wish to consult some of these (e.g., Brinton & Fujiki, 1989; Gallagher, 1991; Lund & Duchan, 1993).

In our own work, we have focused on three major aspects of conversational management; turn exchange, topic manipulation, and conversational repair mechanisms (Brinton & Fujiki, 1989). These particular behaviors were selected because they are generic—they are always present in conversation and as such are essential (Schegloff, 1988). Additionally, these behaviors can be measured reliably, and they seem amenable to intervention.

In identifying patterns of impairment, specific behaviors are compared with developmental expectations drawn from the literature and from the child's community cohort. In addition, the impact of the problematic behaviors on the child's ability to interact with other individuals within his or her community is considered. Specific goals are selected for intervention based on the patterns that have been observed. In selecting goals, we consider two questions: (1) What is the child ready to learn? and (2) What aspect of the problem hinders communication the most? The first point is important in that the child's ability to learn a particular behavior is likely to be influenced by the interaction of the child's cognitive, social, and linguistic capabilities. The

TABLE 5-1. Screening of Conversational Abilities

---

1. Does the child seem hesitant to talk in interactions with peers as well as with adults?
2. Does the child seem overly intimidated by other speakers? For example, does the child give up turns or topics easily if interrupted?
3. Does the child often interrupt other speakers so that they are not allowed to finish sentences or messages?
4. Does the child frequently respond to questions with single-word or stereotypic utterances?
5. Does the child seem to produce a high proportion of back channel responses in conversation with peers and with adults?
6. Does the child often change the topic in response to a question? (Do not count instances in which the child may be avoiding answering, such as in response to "Who broke this?")
7. Does the child often introduce topics without properly introducing referents? Look for utterances such as "He took my pajamas again," in situations in which the listener would not know who "he" is (it is particularly important to consider developmental constraints here).
8. Does the child rarely contribute to topics that are introduced by others?
9. Does the child often continue with a topic even when another speaker has introduced a different topic?
10. Does the child seem to perseverate on certain topics?
11. Does the child seem to have difficulty grasping the "big picture" in conversation, focusing instead on tangential aspects of topics?
12. Does the child seem to have difficulty making relevant contributions to interactions?
13. Does the child often seem to be one step behind the conversation? For example, does the child tend to respond to questions late or continue with topics that others have left?
14. Do other children seem to have difficulty "following" this child in interaction?
15. When talking with this child, do you do an inordinate amount of "work" to make the interaction successful?
16. Does this child have difficulty responding to feedback such as "huh?," "what?," or "This one?"
17. Does this child have difficulty asking for help when he or she does not understand?
18. Do form–content interactions interfere with communication?
19. Do aspects of speech or language draw attention to the speaking process, distracting from the message?

Based on Brinton and Fujiki, 1989.

second point is important in that an estimate of which behaviors hinder communication the most will help to focus attention on critical needs. As the clinician selects treatment goals, a balance should be drawn between these two considerations. However, for each individual child, it will also be important to consider factors such as motivation, parental preferences, and available treatment resources. After considering these factors, a single goal or several goals may be selected for treatment. It is important that goals do not demand the fragmentation and isolation of behaviors.

It should be noted that even though the focus of assessment may be on conversation, structural components of communication cannot be ignored.

Form and content interactions may be assessed as they are used to comprehend and express a variety of communicative functions. Particular attention should be directed to how the phonological, morphological, syntactic, and semantic systems serve the child in conversation.

INTERVENTION WITH CONVERSATIONAL IMPAIRMENT

Speech-language pathologists have traditionally used form–content interactions to support conversation. In other words, the clinician has targeted specific language behaviors, trained those behaviors in limited contexts, and hoped or planned for generalization of those behaviors into conversation as the final stage of intervention. We take a different tack. We use conversation as the primary context for intervention. That is, we use the contextually rich framework available in conversation to support the skills targeted throughout the course of intervention. Conversation is used to support three types of learning. First, conversation supplies the context to facilitate the acquisition of interactional skills. Second, conversation supports the acquisition of structural skills. Third, conversation provides compensatory skills to offset the effects of language difficulties that may persist as the child matures.

When working with conversational parameters, we frequently focus our intervention on turn exchange, topic manipulation, or conversational repair behaviors within certain contexts. However, the primary goal is not to teach turn taking, topic, or repair behaviors per se. Rather, we hope to facilitate these conversational management skills in a way that will enhance communication in a variety of settings that are important to the child. These skills are facilitated by providing enough support in real conversations so that the child's current skills function successfully in interaction. Support for the child's skills can be provided in a number of ways. Factors such as the clinician's input as a conversational partner, the physical setting, the purpose of the interaction, and the addition of conversational participants can all be manipulated to highlight and scaffold the child's contribution.

Before discussing how intervention with conversational impairment might best be approached, it is important to emphasize the importance of the child's conversational partners in the treatment process. Regardless of which procedures are applied, it should be stressed that intervention must include those individuals who interact with the child on a regular basis. Involving parents and caretakers is essential (see MacDonald, 1989). It may also be beneficial to involve teachers, special service providers, and where possible, peers. It has been our experience that when one-half of a dyad demonstrates impairment, both halves show the effect (Fujiki & Brinton, 1991). The child's difficulties in interacting will influence the conversational partner's interactional style as well.

Using patterns of impairment drawn from Fey's (1986) work with conversational responsiveness and assertiveness, some general intervention strategies are outlined as follows.

The inactive communicator.   Fey described the child who is both nonassertive and nonresponsive in conversation as an inactive communicator. This child would be reticent in conversation, infrequently taking turns and rarely initiating topics. The child might also respond only minimally to the bids of the conversational partner.

Working in concert with caretakers and others, the clinician should find the level at which the child is able to successfully take a turn in an exchange and begin intervention at that point. If necessary, the clinician may have to engage the child in nonverbal exchanges. Subsequently, the clinician might imitate the child's behaviors and then make attempts to sustain the interaction in any way feasible. Ideally, intervention would soon progress to entertaining interactive games geared at a level at which the child could participate. For example, for a very young child, activities such as "Peek-a-Boo" or "This Little Piggy" might be appropriate. The response expected from the child would initially be minimal, but it is hoped that the exchange would be rewarding for both partners. For a more mature child, games such as "Go Fish" or "Matching Pairs" could provide a context in which the child is encouraged to take a verbal turn in the interaction. These games could gradually be structured so that more and more is expected from the child.

It will be important to move quickly from structured exchanges, such as games, to less structured interactions, such as guided conversations. As the clinician facilitates the child's participation in guided conversations, manipulation of the context can be a powerful tool. The clinician should try to set up physical contexts and contribute verbal bids that are so inviting that a child will be eager to initiate turns that contribute to a topic. For example, few preschoolers can resist responding to a probe such as "Oh no, look at my shoe!" from a clinician who has just stepped on a fat earthworm. Despite the obvious occupational hazards to clinicians and worms, salient contexts such as this can facilitate the child's appropriate participation in the conversation.

Gradually, the clinician should also support the child's attempts to enter more child-directed conversations. Setting and conversational partners should be carefully varied. Specific techniques to encourage persistence in turn initiation, especially in multispeaker interactions, should be employed. The clinician may integrate topic initiation and maintenance into treatment so that the child will not only take turns, but will also take substantive and appropriate turns. At the same time the clinician is working on turn exchange, ways of improving turn-taking mechanics such as obtaining the listener's attention, anticipating points at which turns will be available, and handling interruptions may also be introduced.

Verbal Noncommunicator. Fey (1986) describes the child who is overly assertive yet nonresponsive to others in conversation as a verbal noncommunicator. Partners engaging in conversations with a nonresponsive child are likely to become less responsive to the child (see Fujiki & Brinton, 1991). Both peers and adults may find conversational interactions with this child difficult.

For this type of child, the intervention plan would be designed to increase responsiveness to listeners. It has been our impression that a high degree of assertiveness in a speaker is acceptable if that speaker is also sensitive to the needs of conversational partners. With regard to turn taking, it may again be necessary to resort to interactive games. In this case, the clinician should highlight giving the turn to another speaker. The clinician may also have to find ways to help this child signal that a turn is available for someone else (such as by using a pause). Turn exchanges may be highlighted by setting up fairly structured interactions in which turn exchange points are overtly marked. For example, the clinician might use a walkie-talkie or radio with which the speaker signals the end of a turn by saying "over."

As a primary focus the clinician should structure conversations so that this child will have to obtain and attend to information provided by another speaker. For example, we might use collaborative games in which different children each conceal part of an important whole such as a puzzle or toy. The child would then need to seek out each child, inquire what the child had, and listen to the response before assembling the whole. As children trade roles in these types of games, they also interact in ways that build cooperative relationships. Another example of an interaction that requires the child to attend to the contributions of others might be ordering from a catalog—the child listens to the requests of others and "takes orders" for goods. We have found that even young preschoolers love these kinds of activities. In summary, the primary lesson that our verbal noncommunicator should learn is that there are better ways to control conversation than to ignore or run over the listener's contributions.

In this discussion we have provided a few examples of methods by which we attempt to "teach" conversation. Obviously, we feel that conversational skills, like other language behaviors, cannot be taught. Rather, they can be facilitated as we present children with situations and provide opportunities for them to make and test hypotheses about how conversations take place.

CASE STUDY

The following case study illustrates some of the principles previously described. J was the fourth of five children from a middle-class, Caucasian family (he had three older brothers and a younger sister). J's parents were concerned that his communication skills were not developing as expected, and at age 4.5

years, he was seen at a children's medical center for psychological and speech-language evaluations. Administration of the *Wechsler Preschool and Primary Scale of Intelligence-Revised* (WPPSI-R) (Wechsler, 1989) produced a verbal IQ of 69, a performance IQ of 105, and a full-scale IQ score of 85. A series of formal measures of speech and language development was administered, all producing scores at least one standard deviation below the mean. J was diagnosed as specifically language-impaired, and it was recommended that he be enrolled in a special classroom for children with language impairment. We began our evaluation of J at the Brigham Young University Speech Language and Hearing Clinic when he was 5.1 years of age. At that time, he was waiting for fall placement in a self-contained, special education kindergarten class for children with a variety of disabilities.

The Screening of Conversational Abilities revealed several areas of concern, including J's ability to respond to questions, his ability to manipulate topics, and his command of form–content interactions. It was decided that an in-depth evaluation including measures of form, content, and conversational management was appropriate.

J appeared to be bright and eager to learn. When engaged in activities that required little language, he could not be distinguished from his peers. However, as soon as language was needed to comprehend, conduct, or mediate an activity, J was at a marked disadvantage. J demonstrated difficulty comprehending complex syntactic forms, recognizing vocabulary, and understanding abstract verbal concepts. In addition, J's productive vocabulary was reduced. Although he produced most of the early developing grammatical morphemes, his production of complex sentence forms was minimal. Attempts to produce complex sentence forms often resulted in structurally incorrect sentences such as "I'm a dad to cook" (for "I'm a dad and I'm cooking" or "I'm a dad who cooks").

In conversation, J seemed adequately assertive with supportive partners. He initiated a fair share of turns in conversation and freely allocated turns to his partners. J initiated topics and typically maintained topics that he initiated. J also maintained topics initiated by others on many occasions. However, topic initiations were generally limited to the current physical context. In other words, J could talk about things that were in front of him, but he had difficulty talking about things that were not present. He frequently failed to respond appropriately to WH questions from his listeners, especially if those questions were explanation questions concerning past or future events. In addition J could not describe or explain a past event clearly.

We were particularly concerned with the way that J managed conversations with his mother and other adults. Adults tended to elicit contributions from J by asking him questions. In response to these questions, J frequently did not respond directly on topic. As a result, adults tended to redirect or rephrase successive questions to J. The more inappropriate J's responses became, the more questions adults tended to ask. The result was a strained interaction described by one adult as "pulling teeth." Consider the following sample:

Child	Mother
	1. What are you going to do when we get home today?
2. Play some my dog.	
	3. Play with your dog?
	4. Wh . . . we don't have a dog.
5. We don't.	
	6. Who you gonna play with?
7. I gonna be, I get, I get a big dog.	
	8. Would you like to get a dog?
9. Yeah, in a pet store.	
	10. In a pet store?
11. A pet store is, where's the pet store?	
	12. What would Rowdy do if you got a dog? [Rowdy is the family cat]
13. I'll get two pets, (2).	
	14. Two pets?
15. Mmm hmm. [yes]	
16. You got (1).	
	17. (1) got Rowdy?
18. Yeah, I pet . . . a this a dog.	
	19. So what are you going to do when you get home today?
	20. Who are you going to play with?
21. My doggy.	
	22. Who else?
23. (laughs) No.	
	24. Hmmm?
25. He's got a hamburger.	
	26. Hamburger?
27. Mmm, a (3)	
	28. Are you gonna play with Hillary?
29. No.	
	30. No?
	31. Are you gonna play with Julia?
32. No.	
	33. Are you gonna play with Nathan?
34. No.	
	35. Are you gonna play with Jesse?
36. Yeah!	

Comments of the transcriber are in brackets; unintelligible sequences are in parentheses with the number of unintelligible syllables indicated.

In choosing treatment goals for J, we first considered what he was ready to learn cognitively and linguistically. Since J's nonverbal functioning was within normal limits, we were not hampered by cognitive constraints. Linguistically, J seemed ready to learn many skills a step advanced from his current level. Possible areas to work on included lexical items, specific morphological forms, complex sentence forms, abstract verbal concepts, and manipulation of decontextualized topics. In considering what would bolster J's communication system the most, we were impressed by the effect that J's communication skills had on his interactions with his mother. It seemed that the more his mother tried to "teach," the more difficult her interaction with J became.

We decided to concentrate on several goals. These included (1) improving topic maintenance within question–answer sequences, (2) increasing the ability to discuss topics drawn from past and future events, (3) increasing available lexical items, and (4) increasing the ability to map two or more ideas onto a single complex sentence form. All of these goals were addressed simultaneously within the context of conversation.

A three-pronged service delivery model was implemented. First, our clinician worked with J on a one-to-one basis in the university clinic setting. Second, we worked with J's mother, focusing on her interaction with J at home and in the clinic. Third, we worked with J's special education classroom teacher and speech-language pathologist at school. Jay was seen twice a week in the clinic. We saw his mother during those times and we had phone contact with her at other times as well. Contact with the school was less frequent and more formal, taking place in the course of meetings and phone contacts during the school year.

In order to increase J's ability to maintain a topic appropriately in question–answer sequences, our first objective was to decrease the number of questions that adults asked him. Special attention was directed toward monitoring our input, as well as working with J's mother to adjust her input. J's mother was quick to appreciate that her series of questions usually had a negative result. However, we made no attempt to eliminate questions altogether. Rather, didactic or test questions were eliminated, leaving only those questions to which J could contribute a response that contained information previously unavailable to the adult. In other words, we eliminated questions to which we already knew the answer (e.g., "What did we do yesterday?") in favor of questions that really mattered (e.g., "What do you want for dessert?"). We suggested a number of interactional strategies to J's mother that could substitute for the series of test questions she had been using. For example, she was encouraged to follow J's lead, to expand J's utterances, to ground her explanations in the current context, and to initiate and develop topics of interest to J. Similar interactional strategies were suggested to J's teacher and speech-language pathologist.

In order to encourage J to initiate and develop topics that were not dependent on the current physical context, attention was concentrated on describing past and future events. Events with salient components were set up (such as a shopping trip to the grocery store where the clinician dropped a bag of groceries). Later in the intervention session, a discussion of these events was initiated. In addition, the clinician familiarized herself with past or planned events in J's homelife and encouraged J to discuss these events. J's mother regularly helped him select objects or materials that were important to him to bring to the intervention session. These objects were used as "springboards" for discussion of events that occurred outside of the clinic.

In working with J's lexical development, lexical items were presented within topical themes in a conversational context. For example, the clinician set up a grocery store in the clinic room. J and his clinician then made a list of items to buy and drew them on a chalkboard. They went to the store they had set up to purchase the items. The clinician pointed and named various items in categories, noting their attributes and similarities and differences. J selected items from his list. The clinician followed J's lead as he pretended to take the items home and shelve them with like items. Several unfamiliar items were mixed with familiar ones. These new items were always presented within familiar categories. J's mother watched and sometimes participated in activities. She soon adapted these methods to use at home during her daily routine. For example, she enlisted J's help to fix dinner. She described items they would need, noting functions and similarities and differences. She tried to keep her input clear and interesting, while being responsive to J's contributions.

J's teacher and speech-language pathologist were encouraged to present lexical items and language-based concepts in a way that would make them as salient to J as possible. We asked for copies of lesson plans so that lexical items important to Jay's academic work could be incorporated into our clinical intervention. In working with J's school, the most difficult obstacle encountered was the fact that his academic curriculum was rapid and fragmented. For instance, one week the teacher introduced the concept of community helpers, the next week she moved to body parts, and the next week it was on Halloween activities. New concepts and lexical items were presented much too rapidly and without sufficient depth to fit J's learning style. It was suggested that J's learning would be maximized if he worked within theme areas that were developed in more detail (Norris & Damico, 1990). It was also suggested that concepts be presented within overriding content areas or curricular units that provided multiple opportunities for J to discover new meanings.

In approaching J's mapping of multiple ideas onto single complex sentence forms, a focused stimulation approach was used (Fey, 1986). Within conversation, complex sentences were presented to express ideas important in that setting. We concentrated on forms that expressed cause and effect or means to an end. These forms were highlighted using stress and intonation. The clinician also expanded some of J's simple forms into complex forms. For example, while grocery shopping, the clinician would model forms such as "I need a bag so I can carry the groceries," or "We'll open this box to see what's inside." If J said something like "This is good. I buy this," the clinician would model, "That is good, so we'll buy it."

The most immediate result of intervention with J was a change in his conversational interactions with his mother. The number of didactic questions directed to J decreased. Additionally, J's mother attempted to follow J's lead more often and concentrated on modeling forms and lexical items in meaningful interactions. Despite the increased monitoring required in her interactions with J, she reported that their conversations became much "easier" for her. She found it much more rewarding and satisfying to converse with her son. She felt that he was contributing much more appropriate, topical information to their interactions, and she happily noted the emergence of complex sentence forms on some occasions. By the same token, we felt that she had become a better facilitator of J's communication skills.

Transcripts of clinical sessions indicated that maintenance of topic in response to WH questions improved. This was, in part, a function of the fact that there were fewer questions directed at him than had previously been the case. J did not appear to have so much trouble fielding simple, meaningful questions.

Discussing topics that revolved around past and future events continued to be difficult for J. However, he experienced considerable success discussing past and future events that were linked to the present context by materials he brought into the clinic.

As we worked with J, instances were noted in which he evidently did not know or could not retrieve lexical items. Where appropriate, these items were then incorporated into treatment. For example, it became clear that J could not name a piece of chalk or a napkin. On another occasion his mother reported that he did not recognize the word "drawer." These and other similarly identified items were incorporated into future interactions.

J also began to produce a high frequency of related utterances that appeared to be steps to the appropriate formation of complex sentences. He produced utterances such as "I need a hammer. I can pound this" which lacked only a conjunction to indicate the link in ideas. Previously, many of his complex sentences were ill formed and difficult to interpret.

In summary, the most effective aspect of intervention with J was improving his conversational interactions with adults. This resulted not only from improvement in J's abilities but also because his mother and clinician provided better support. The result was a more supportive interaction in which J's language learning could be facilitated. J's use of language structure within conversations continued to develop. It became easier to talk with him, and to understand his intent. We could demonstrate improvement in his ability to manage conversations that incorporated a variety of developing linguistic structures.

NOTE

The authors would like to thank J and his mother for permission to report J's case. We would also like to acknowledge the work of Lee Robinson, our research assistant, and the support of the undergraduate research trainee program at Brigham Young University.

REFERENCES

Brinton, B, & Fujiki, M. (1989). *Conversational management with language-impaired children: Pragmatic assessment and intervention.* Rockville, MD: Aspen.

Duchan, J. (1984). Language assessment: The pragmatics revolution. In R. Naremore (Ed.), *Language science.* San Diego, CA: College-Hill Press.

Fey, M. (1986). *Language intervention wtih young children.* San Diego, CA: College-Hill Press.

Fujiki, M., & Brinton, B. (1991). The verbal noncommunicator: A case study. *Language, Speech and Hearing Services in Schools, 22,* 322–333.

Gallagher, T.M. (1991). A retrospective look at clinical pragmatics. In T.M. Gallagher, (Ed.), *Pragmatics of language: Clinical practice issues.* San Diego, CA: Singular Publishing Group.

Lund, N., & Duchan, J., (1993). *Assessing children's language in naturalistic contexts* (3rd ed.). Englewood Cliffs, NJ.: Prentice Hall.

MacDonald, J.D. (1989). *Becoming partners with children: From play to conversation.* San Antonio, TX: Special Press, Inc.

Norris, J., & Damico, J. (1990). Whole language in theory and practice: Implications for language intervention. *Language, Speech and Hearing Services in Schools, 21,* 212–220.

Schegloff, E. (1988). *Other-initiated repair sequences in talk in interaction.* Successful grant proposal, National Science Foundation.

Van Riper, C. (1939). *Speech correction: Principles and methods.* Englewood Cliffs, NJ: Prentice Hall.

Wechsler, D. (1989). *Wechsler Preschool and Primary Scale of Intelligence–Revised.* San Antonio: Psychological Corporation.

chapter 6

CHILDREN'S DEVELOPING NOTIONS OF OTHERS' MINDS

Janet Wilde Astington

An idea that threads through the chapters in this book is that scripts, narratives, and stories help children to make sense of the world. Indeed, narrative helps us all to make sense of the world (Bruner, 1986). But what is it that we, and children, are trying to make sense of? It's not just the physical world—much of the time it's the social world: other people, and our interactions with them. What we care about, what we want to understand, is what people are doing, how that fits in with what we are going to do, how it will affect others, and so on. When we talk about these things, we want to know *why* people did what they did, and we want to be able to tell what they are going to do next.

This might make us sound like psychologists and that is just what I intend. Psychologists try to explain why people act the way they do and try to predict what people will do. In that sense, we are all psychologists. We are all interested in the things people do: "Why did she do that?" "What will he do next?" This is the way we talk all the time. Now, psychologists' explanations depend on the particular theory they hold. Behaviorists say things like, "She has been reinforced for producing that behavior in the past." Neuropsychologists say things like, "Neuron #529 is firing"—perhaps that is too much of a caricature, but their interest is in how brain activity underlies behavior. The question is: What do we do, not in the lab but in our ordinary lives? How do we talk about these things in our everyday conversations? We say things like, "She did it because she *wanted* it." "I looked in there because that's where I *thought* it was." "He *felt* sad and so he went away." That is, we talk about what people think, and want, and feel.

Even five-year-olds talk like this. We need only listen to them, or look in Vivian Paley's books, to see that they, too, do it all the time. Here, Paley is talking to the children about a story she has just read to them:

Teacher: Why was she [Goldilocks] in the woods?

Mary Anne: Maybe she was looking for blackberries and she thought this was the way she always went through the woods, but it wasn't.

Clarice: What if she thinks it's her own house?

Charlotte: She did think it's her own house. She probably has the same furniture.

(Paley, 1984, pp. 51–52)

Here's another example:

Teacher: Why does Jack decide to climb the beanstalk?

Charlotte: He wants to find out what was up there.

Mary Anne: Maybe he thinks it's very cloudy up there and he doesn't know if there's a king or a giant up there to rest.

Jill: Maybe he thinks they're rich up there and there's lots of food.

Teacher: Why does the giant's wife help Jack?

Karen: She likes little boys. She doesn't want the giant to eat him.

(Paley, 1984, p. 59)

The children's responses are rich in mental language. They refer to what the story characters think and know and want and feel. Of course, the children are helped by Paley's "why" questions. This helps to produce exactly the sort of child-involved analytical talk David Dickinson discusses in his chapter, talk that is rich in mental language. We not only use this sort of language to talk about stories, and what story characters do, we use it to justify and explain our own behavior as well. And so do the five-year-olds, so does Wally, for example. Paley is playing a guessing game with the kindergarten children to see what they understand of probability. Ten red cards and two blue ones are placed face down and mixed up. The child has to guess the color of a card before turning it over.

Wally predicted blue every time, yet he always turned up a red square. I asked, "Why do you keep choosing blue when there are so many reds and only two blues?" "I know that," Wally answered. "I just want blue to come up. I'm wishing for it to come up."

(Paley, 1981, p. 80)

Thus, in general, we explain and predict our own and others' actions by referring to mental states, to our own and others' beliefs, desires, intentions, and emotions. This is what is known as *folk psychology,* because it is the psychology ordinary folk use. It may be referred to as *commonsense psychology,* because it is, after all, common sense. It is also often referred to as *belief–desire psychology,* because that is what it appeals to—people's beliefs and desires, what they think and want. We assume people will act in a way that will satisfy their desires, given their beliefs.

Here is another example of this kind of thinking. A colleague rushes past me in the hall. Why did Jenny race past me without stopping to talk?—Because she thought it was nine o'clock and she wanted to get to her meeting on time. When we know what someone believes and desires, we can predict what that person will do. There are three basic considerations—belief, desire, and action; given any two of these we can work out the third one. If we know Jenny wants to be on time and that she thinks she's late, we can predict that she'll hurry past us. If we see her race by and we know she wants to get to the meeting on time, we explain her action by saying she must think she's late. And if she rushes by, crying "I'm late!," we know she wants to be on time. We also talk about people's emotions and intentions. Jenny was ashamed she'd been late every week so far and she intended to do better this week. That is, in order to explain and predict someone's actions we refer to his or her beliefs, desires, emotions, and intentions. Believing it's late, desiring to be on time, and being ashamed of always being late, intending to improve—these are all states of mind. In fact, mental states, all of our thoughts, wants, feelings, plans, together *are* our mind.

As children start to understand and talk about what people think, and want, and feel, so they develop their notions about the mind, about their own mind, and about other people's minds. This topic has become a lively area of research in child development in the last few years. The field is known as *children's theory of mind* (Astington, Harris, & Olson, 1988). Although it is referred to as a "theory" of mind, there is a lot of argument about whether folk psychology really is a theory, that is, whether children's notions of mind are acquired by theory construction or in some other way (Astington & Gopnik, 1991b). Nonetheless, those who argue that folk psychology is not a theory still identify this research area as the study of children's theory of mind.

I have three aims in this chapter. First, I discuss the history and background of this new research area. Second, I review the research findings in the area, what we know about children's notions of mind. And third, I consider how this work relates to the general concern of this volume; that is, I discuss the relation between pragmatics and children's theory of mind.

HISTORY AND BACKGROUND OF RESEARCH IN CHILDREN'S THEORY OF MIND

This area of research has developed from a number of sources. It is an area that provides a meeting point for different branches of developmental psychology: cognitive, social, and linguistic. It also draws on work in the philosophy of mind, and on work in animal psychology.

In fact the phrase "theory of mind" was first used in this context in a report of a lab study of chimpanzees by David Premack and Guy Woodruff (1978) called, "Does the chimpanzee have a theory of mind?" These two psychologists were interested in the chimpanzee's ability to predict human action. They showed the chimp videotapes of a human actor faced with a problem, such as bananas out of reach, hanging from the ceiling. They stopped the videotape and gave the chimp two photographs. One was a "solution" to the problem; for example, it showed the actor climbing onto a box. The chimpanzee's task was to choose one of the two photographs. Premack and Woodruff showed that the chimp usually chose the photograph of the problem solution. They claimed that this showed that the chimpanzee had a "theory of mind," which they defined in the following way:

> An individual has a theory of mind if he imputes mental states to himself and others. A system of inferences of this kind is properly viewed as a theory because such states are not directly observable, and the system can be used to make predictions about the behavior of others.

> (Premack & Woodruff, 1978, p. 515)

That is, the chimpanzee attributed an unseen mental state to the actor (wanting to get the bananas) and used it to make predictions about his action (he would climb on the box). Premack and Woodruff called it a "theory" because the mental state was not observable and was used to make a behavioral prediction.

Developmentalists took up the term "theory of mind" and Premack and Woodruff's definition of it and applied it to typical children (Bretherton, McNew, & Beeghly-Smith, 1981; Wellman, 1985) and atypical children (especially autistic children—see Hewitt, Chapter 7, and Leslie, 1991). A philosophical debate regarding Premack and Woodruff's claims also ensued. Three different philosophers (Bennett, 1978; Dennett, 1978; Harman, 1978) described the paradigmatic experiment that they each said would be needed to show that someone or some animal possessed a theory of mind—a basic test that would show that someone attributed mental states to another person.

Their proposals led to an experiment by two developmental psychologists, Heinz Wimmer and Josef Perner (1983). They designed a task that uses "false belief" stories acted out for the child with dolls and toys. One story goes like this (Perner, Leekam, & Wimmer, 1987): A boy and his mother come home from the store with a bag of shopping. The boy has bought some chocolate; he puts it in a drawer and goes out to play. Later his mother uses some of the chocolate to make a cake, and when she's finished she puts the chocolate back into a cupboard, not into the drawer. Then she goes off upstairs. Then the boy comes back inside, hungry and wanting his chocolate.

The crucial question is, "Where will the boy look for the chocolate?" It is obvious to us that he will look in the drawer. We would not be surprised to see him look there, and we would not be surprised when he doesn't find chocolate there. This is simple but very important. Our lack of surprise demonstrates two fundamental aspects of our way of thinking. First, we believe there is a real world out there, which includes real objects such as chocolates and drawers and cupboards. These real things exist quite independently of our thoughts about them. But second, we believe we do have thoughts about these things, and sometimes those thoughts do not reflect the way things really are in the world. Nonetheless, in that case we act, not on the basis of the way things really are, but on the basis of the way we think they are. That is to say, our relationship to the world is mediated by mental representations.

These two beliefs are so deep-rooted in our way of thinking, it is almost impossible for us to imagine what it would be like not to have them, not to think in that way. But have we always had them? What if we acted out this story for a three-year-old. What would the three-year-old say? She would say that the boy would look in the cupboard (Perner et al., 1987). We could ask her questions that made it quite clear that she knew that the boy put the chocolate in the drawer in the beginning, and then he went outside, and he wasn't there when his mother moved it, and he didn't see her move it. But even so, when we ask the three-year-old where the boy will look, she says that he will look in the cupboard. He will look there because he wants his chocolate, and that is where his chocolate is. The three-year-old understands that people act on the basis of their desires, on what they want. However, she does not understand that people also act on the basis of their beliefs, on the way they think things are, not on the basis of the way things really are.

What if we ask a four-year-old? She will tell us that the boy will look in the drawer. The only way the child can give this answer is by attributing a *false belief* to the boy. The child has to understand that what the boy believes is different from what she knows to be the case. There is no other way of predicting the boy's action correctly. Children who make this correct prediction are able to attribute mental states to others—they have notions of others' minds, a theory of mind. Children first acquire this understanding at about four years of age.

Children's theory of mind research has roots in laboratory studies of animal behavior, and also in studies of naturally occurring behavior, such as the primate's ability to practice deception (Mitchell & Thompson, 1986). Intelligent primates have been called "natural psychologists" because of the way they manipulate other members of their social group. This might suggest that intelligence has evolved to handle the problems of social life (Byrne & Whiten, 1988).

Work in theory of mind also draws on philosophical theories of intentionality, and the technical concept of mental representation. Mental states are called *intentional states,* not in the everyday sense of "on purpose," but in the philosophical sense (Brentano, 1960)—intentional states are mental states that are *about* things (Dennett, 1987). A mental state consists of an attitude and a content. The attitude is the kind of mental state that it is— belief, desire, intention, and so on. The content is what it is about—something or some event in the world, or some nonexistent thing or event, for example, "He believes it's snowing," "She wants Santa Claus to come." Even infants have mental states such as beliefs, desires, and intentions. But this is a different issue from having notions about mental states and being able to attribute them to other people, as in the false belief task.

Beyond its links with philosophy and animal psychology, work in children's theory of mind unites a number of different areas of developmental psychology. Research in social cognition is obviously of relevance to children's theory of mind, since it concerns children's perception of others, their understanding of others, and their role-taking ability. This goes all the way back to Piaget's early work and the concept of egocentrism (Piaget, 1924/1928). Another area of research in cognitive development is also relevant here— children's metacognition. This concerns children's knowledge of cognitive processes, especially their own mental processes in school-like settings. What is different about research on children's theory of mind is that developmentalists no longer think of social cognition and metacognition as separate research areas. Rather, they consider that children are acquiring a coherent body of knowledge—understanding other people's minds and their own mind. For instance, it is not simply that preschoolers do not understand what other people think, they do not understand their own minds either, and they develop both social knowledge and metaknowledge together.

In the early 1980s, at the beginning of research into children's theory of mind, the focus was on experimental work in cognitive development. Not much attention was paid to the social context. Developmentalists, Judy Dunn (1988) especially, pointed to a paradox. Four-year-olds could be said to understand others' minds, based on their performance on experimental tasks such as the false belief task, but three-year-olds could not. However, as any parent knows, and as all Dunn's observations showed, two- and three-year-olds are competent participants in social interactions. They seem to understand and to be able to manipulate their family members' intentions and emotions. Thus, the social context underlying children's understanding of emotion was brought into theory of mind research. In addition, research into language development, especially pragmatic development, was included in attempts to understand children's developing notions of others' minds (e.g., Bruner, 1983).

All these different fields—animal psychology; philosophy of mind; and cognitive, social, and linguistic developmental studies—have fed into theory of mind research. The field offers challenging problems with important real-world implications. It addresses fundamental issues—what makes us human and how we understand ourselves and others. Even if we do not want to think of this development as children's theory acquisition and prefer the more neutral term folk psychology, it is still a vital development, in need of explanation and having real implications for social behavior.

REVIEW OF RESEARCH FINDINGS

What do children of different ages understand about people's minds? Tied to this question is: What will count as evidence? It is important to note that we are not looking for verbalizable understanding of mind of the kind professional philosophers and psychologists have, or even of the kind that can be obtained by conducting interviews with children (Broughton, 1978). We are concerned with the sort of understanding that can be inferred from what children say and do. It is the sort of understanding that is shown in our everyday interactions with each other—the ways in which we explain why we did something, and the ways in which we predict what our friends will do. In other words, it is our folk psychological understanding of how actions are guided and motivated by beliefs and desires. I focus here on research studies of typical children from Western cultures, in the years between two and five, and primarily on work in cognitive development, because that is where theory of mind research has been concentrated. Even then, there are about two hundred relevant articles. The papers I cite are selected for their representativeness. A more detailed review can be found in Astington (1993).

The research has been conducted almost entirely in Western settings. There are very little cross-cultural data available. Some data suggest that children universally develop similar notions about the mind (Avis & Harris, 1991), whereas other data suggest that children's understanding depends on the particular social and linguistic environment in which they grow up (McCormick, 1990). There may be an element of truth to both suggestions. There may be a universal core to the understanding of mind, differently modulated in different societies (Harris, 1990).

There has been little direct work on infants' notions of mind. Infants readily engage in social interaction. They smile, make eye contact, coo, babble, gesture to be picked up and to be given things, offer things, look where another person looks, and so on. Clearly they distinguish between people and objects, attributing agency to people, not to objects (Stern, 1985). However, although these behaviors reflect social understandings, they should not necessarily be interpreted as indicative of infants' explicit understanding of other people's minds.

Things change at the end of infancy, at about eighteen months of age, with the development of symbolic abilities. Children's pretend play, which begins at this age—their ability to pretend and to enter into pretend play with others, shows that they can reason about hypothetical situations, a skill central to the development of their understanding of their own and others' minds (Leslie, 1988). For example, when a two-year-old picks up a banana and talks into it as if it were a telephone, he can see it in one way (as a banana) and think about it in another way (as a telephone).

After two years of age children start to talk about their own and other people's perceptions, desires, and emotions, about what they themselves and others see, look at, taste, like, love, want, are happy about, feel sad about, and so on (Bretherton & Beeghly, 1982). By three, children refer to cognitive states as well. They talk about what they and others know, think, remember, and so on. It is important to look at more than simply the child's use of a mental term, which may be merely idiomatic, as when a child says "Know what?" to introduce a new topic. We need to look at the child's ability to use these words to refer to people's mental states, and to contrast mental states with reality. Three-year-old children can make such contrasts (Shatz, Wellman, & Silber, 1983).

Two- and three-year-olds show that they understand something about perception, desire, and emotion in experimental tasks too. They can produce perceptions in others and deprive others of perception by showing and hiding things (Lempers, Flavell, & Flavell, 1977). By three they can also judge another's perception or lack of it in other modalities as well as sight—hearing, smell, and touch (Yaniv & Shatz, 1988). Two- and three-year-olds understand something about how desires may determine actions and emotions. For example, if they are told what a story character wants, they can predict what he will do (Wellman & Woolley, 1990). They can judge emotional reactions in a similar way, as indicated by their ability to judge that people are happy if they get what they want, and sad if they don't.

After three years of age children show a more explicit understanding of the mind. Three-year-olds can distinguish between real and mental entities (Wellman & Estes, 1986). For example, if they are told one boy has a cookie and another boy is thinking about a cookie, they can tell you which cookie can be eaten, shared, and so on. And they can explicitly distinguish between pretense and reality (Flavell, Flavell, & Green, 1987). Three-year-olds also have a more explicit understanding of the links between perception and knowledge and can recognize that if an object is hidden in a box, someone who has looked in the box will know what is in there, and someone who has not looked will not know (Pratt & Bryant, 1990).

Like two-year-olds, three-year-olds can predict a person's actions based on what the person wants. Moreover, they can predict a person's actions based on what the person thinks, so long as what the other thinks does not conflict with what the child actually knows to be the case (Wellman & Bartsch, 1988). Three-year-olds also understand something about intentions. In simple ways they can distinguish between intended and unintended actions. They talk about things being done on purpose, and they recognize that people are pleased when their intentions are fulfilled (Astington, 1991).

Despite all these achievements, there are a lot of things that three-year-olds cannot do that four-year-olds can. The most famous of these is the ability to predict someone's actions when he or she holds a false belief. When typical three-year-olds are asked where a boy will look for a hidden chocolate that has been moved from the place where he last saw it, most predict that he will look in the new place, where the chocolate actually is. They do not seem to understand that the boy will look for it where he thinks it is, in the old place.

In its original form this task was quite hard even for four-year-olds (Wimmer & Perner, 1983), but when the task was simplified, and the salient features made extremely clear, four-year-olds could answer correctly, but three-year-olds could not (Perner et al., 1987). They have difficulty even when given considerable contextual support, as when they are shown the story on videotape, with the actor actually looking in the old place, where he thinks the object is, and expressing surprise when he finds an unexpected object (Moses & Flavell, 1990).

Three-year-olds' difficulty understanding false belief is apparent in situations involving unexpected contents, not just those involving unexpected locations. Three-year-olds shown a familiar candy box and allowed to discover that there are pencils rather than candy inside cannot determine that a friend who has not seen inside the box will think candy is inside it. Most say the friend will think there are pencils in the box (Perner et al., 1987). Furthermore, it is not just false belief in others that is hard for three-year-olds to understand. They do not understand it in themselves either. They do not recognize that their beliefs change when they find out they were wrong. If the child is asked what she thought was in the box when she first saw it, she will say she thought there were pencils inside it, not candy, even though she may have said "candy" a minute earlier (Gopnik & Astington, 1988).

From the Piagetian perspective of egocentrism, a three-year-old responds that the other child will think there are pencils in the candy box because that is what she knows to be in there. She does not understand how others can have beliefs different from her own. However, the child's response involves more than mere egocentricity. She does not understand her own mind either. She does not understand that she used to think something that she now knows is not the case. Furthermore, she comes to understand both these things at the same time. It is not that she understands herself and then applies that to other people—the old Cartesian argument. She acquires a coherent body of knowledge about the mind—her own mind and other people's minds—all at one time.

Just as three-year-olds do not understand how someone can believe something different from what they know is really the case, they do not understand how something can look different from what it really is. They do not understand, for example, that a joke-store "rock" looks like a rock but is really a sponge, whereas four-year-olds do (Flavell, 1986). Once three-year-olds find out the object is really a sponge, they say it looks like a sponge.

Three-year-olds understand that a person who has looked in a box knows what is in there and someone who has not looked does not know, but they do not understand that two people may have different views of the same thing. For example, if a picture is put on the table between two people, so that one of them sees it the right way up and the other sees it upside down, four-year-olds understand the discrepancy but three-year-olds do not (Flavell, Everett, Croft, & Flavell, 1981). Nor do three-year-olds understand that people may acquire different information from the same perceptual experience (Ruffman, Olson, & Astington, 1991). Four-year-olds understand that what you know about an object depends on the sensory modality that is involved; that is, you have to see an object to know its color, but you have to feel it to know its texture (O'Neill, Astington, & Flavell, 1992). Three-year-olds do not understand this, although they can, of course, get information via these different senses.

In addition, there are things about intention and desire that three-year-olds do not understand that the older children do (Astington & Gopnik, 1991a). Three-year-olds do not understand the causal link between intention and action, and they do not focus on the future-directedness of intention. They cannot predict action based on desire if they have to infer a desire that conflicts with their own desire. The older children succeed on these tasks. And by five children start to understand more complex cognitive emotions like surprise, and they understand the dependence of emotion on belief— that is, we are happy if we think we're getting what we want (Harris, 1989). Children of this age also understand the relative certainty expressed by *know* over *think* and *must* over *might* (Moore, Pure, & Furrow, 1990).

The important point about the wide range of abilities I have discussed is that many of them are correlated. That is, regardless of age, individual children come to understand many of these things at the same time. Experimental work has demonstrated correlations between children's understanding of others' false beliefs, of their own earlier false beliefs, their understanding of the distinction between appearance and reality, and their comprehension of expressions of relative certainty (Gopnik & Astington, 1988; Moore et al., 1990). Many researchers have argued that this indicates some underlying conceptual change, indicative of children's development of a theory of mind (Astington, 1993).

This brief review shows that there is enormous development in children's understanding of the mind in the years between two and five. However, even at five children are not like adults. There is still considerable development in the understanding of the mind during the school years—in metacognition; understanding personality traits; understanding embedded mental states such as beliefs about beliefs, and the social concepts that depend on them, such as responsibility, foreseeability, commitment, reliance, deception, and so on. There is also development in children's understanding of the expression of these concepts in speech acts, promising, lying, irony and so on—that is, in their understanding of pragmatics. It is the relation between pragmatics and theory of mind to which I now turn.

PRAGMATICS AND THEORY OF MIND

How does this work on children's understanding of mind relate to pragmatics? Theory of mind has been such a lively field in the last few years, with new studies appearing all the time. Some people have asked what is new about theory of mind. Isn't it a new name for the kind of investigations that have been going on for a long time, in social cognition, for example? I think that theory of mind is much more than an old field with a new name. It draws on and synthesizes a number of different areas of investigation and presents new views on old problems; for example, I mentioned the new view on egocentrism—that young children are not egocentric but come to understand their own mind and other people's minds at one and the same time.

Now that the first flurries of excitement have died down, there are important questions to ask about the relation of children's theory of mind to other aspects of development, aspects that also depend on an understanding of people's beliefs, desires, intentions, and emotions. Pragmatics is one of these areas. When we begin to think about the relation between children's pragmatic ability and their understanding of others' minds, we are faced with something of a puzzle. Obviously there must be some relation between the two, since both do involve an appreciation of others' beliefs and intentions, but the timing seems wrong in some way. Children's pragmatic understanding precedes by a few years their understanding of other people's minds, at least that aspect of theory of mind shown by successful performance on false belief tasks.

However, maybe one should say it is their pragmatic *ability* that precedes their understanding of others' minds, not their pragmatic *understanding*. There is an important difference here. Perhaps there is some implicit sort of understanding expressed in pragmatic ability, as Bretherton and her colleagues proposed (Bretherton et al., 1981). Certainly, from early on, even before they talk, children participate in social interaction, and social interaction requires that mental states be communicated to others. We have to let the other person know that we want something, or that we want to believe something. Human beings are not mindreaders, at least not in any telepathic sense. In order to know what is in the other person's mind we have to give that information to one another. We have to "get in touch" and "get it across." This is the communication that is basic to social interaction. It frequently, although not exclusively, involves language. You have your beliefs, desires, and so on, and I have mine. We share these in language, in the talk that passes between us.

The basic notion of *speech act theory* (Searle, 1969) is that communicating mental states involves expressing them as speech acts. The propositional content of the mental state becomes the propositional content of the speech act. Just as I believe that John stole the money, I can swear that John stole the money (Astington, 1990b). Just as I can want you to come to my party, I can ask you to come to my party. Just as I can intend to mow the lawn, I can promise to mow the lawn. Emotions too are expressed in speech acts: regret in apologies, gratitude in thanks, and so on. Even infants have such mental states—they have beliefs, desires, and intentions. We can see their surprise when something unexpected happens, when their belief is not confirmed. And we can see their rage when a desire is frustrated. Moreover, their communication appears to be intentional. If a baby wants something and the parent does not respond, the baby looks back at the parent, looks at the object again, adds a sound to his reaching gesture, makes it louder, and so on, until there is some response from the parent (Lock, 1978, 1980). Certainly the infant's behavior appears intentional.

However, having beliefs, desires, and intentions is not the same as understanding about belief, desire, and intention and being able to attribute those states to others. At this stage it is hard to say how much infants really understand about people's minds. Bretherton et al. (1981), more than ten years ago now, suggested that infants' ability to communicate with others shows that they have a theory of mind. Nonetheless they were not suggesting that infants could impute *mental* states to others. Infants have an *implicit* theory of mind, they said, in the same way that two-year-olds have an implicit theory of grammar (Bretherton et al., 1981, p. 340). Even so, infants do respond to other people's expressions of belief and desire. Mother says, "There's a truck," points, and the baby looks. Father says, "Give me the ball," holds out his hand, and the baby gives it. Infants are active participants in the social exchange. The crucial question is, how much understanding do they have of it?

I think perhaps that just as children's theory of mind is marked by their understanding of mental states, not merely possession of them, so the analogous development in pragmatics is metapragmatic understanding. That is, it is not the production of speech acts—statements, requests, and so on. It is not even the interpretation of other people's statements and requests. It is metapragmatic understanding. In Chapter 12, Catherine Snow describes metapragmatics as being tuned in to the rules, not just simply focused on the conversation. The informal and formal definitions that she describes children giving are equally communicative, but the child who produces a formal definition has analyzed the pragmatic demands of the situation. It would be interesting to see whether that is a skill that correlates with theory of mind abilities.

We also see this metapragmatic skill in children's ability to judge the appropriateness of speech acts, for example, their judgments of requests, their ability to recognize indirectness (Bates, 1976). We see it too in children's understanding of the pragmatic rules governing promising (Astington, 1990a). Metapragmatic understanding may also be involved in lying, at least deliberate lying, and understanding that other people are lying. These are developments that do not come until about four years of age (Leekam, 1991). Younger children can produce speech acts that we may call lies, but they do not understand them *as* lies; they do not recognize the point or purpose of a lie. They do know how to manipulate situations, but they do not know how to manipulate people's beliefs about situations. Joan Peskin (1992, p. 84) has an appropriate anecdote that illustrates this, from when her son was three years old:

Child: Mommy, Go out of the kitchen.

Mother: Why?

Child: Because I want to take a cookie.

The child knows that he needs to manipulate the mother's behavior, but he does not understand that it is in order to affect her beliefs.

In conclusion: What is currently needed in theory of mind research is an integration of the relevant cognitive, social, and linguistic data. Attempts to work out the relations between pragmatics and children's understanding of mind may be the best way of getting to that. Pragmatics involves the linguistic production, in a social situation, of propositional content that depends on a cognitive understanding of the participants, of their intentions and interpretations. Thus, studying language as a communication system, being concerned with children's developing use of language, puts one in a good position to understand children's developing notions of others' minds. And, as Lynne Hewitt (Chapter 7) suggests, being aware of the impact of communicative competence of these developing notions of mind will, in turn, enhance understanding of language development and disorders.

NOTE

I am grateful to the Spencer Foundation and to the Natural Sciences and Engineering Research Council of Canada for financial support.

REFERENCES

Astington, J. W. (1990a). Metapragmatics: Children's conception of promising. In G. Conti-Ramsden & C. Snow (Eds.), *Children's language* (pp. 223–244). Hillsdale, NJ: Lawrence Erlbaum.

Astington, J. W. (1990b). Narrative and the child's theory of mind. In B. Britton & A. Pellegrini (Eds.). *Narrative thought and narrative language* (pp. 151–171). Hillsdale, NJ: Lawrence Erlbaum.

Astington, J. W. (1991). Intention in the child's theory of mind. In D. Frye & C. Moore (Eds.). *Children's theories of mind* (pp. 157–172). Hillsdale, NJ: Lawrence Erlbaum.

Astington, J. W. (1993). *The child's discovery of the mind.* Cambridge, MA: Harvard University Press.

Astington, J. W., & Gopnik, A. (1991a). Developing understanding of desire and intention. In A. Whiten (Ed.). *Natural theories of mind: Evolution, development and stimulation of everyday mindreading* (pp. 39–50). Oxford: Basil Blackwell.

Astington, J. W., & Gopnik, A. (1991b). Theoretical explanations of children's understanding of the mind. *British Journal of Developmental Psychology, 9,* 7–31.

Astington, J. W., Harris, P. L., & Olson, D. R. (Eds.). (1988). *Developing theories of mind.* New York: Cambridge University Press.

Avis, J., & Harris, P. L. (1991). Belief–desire reasoning among Baka children: Evidence for a universal conception of mind. *Child Development, 62,* 460–467.

Bates, E. (1976). *Language and context: The acquisition of pragmatics.* New York: Academic Press.

Bennett, J. (1978). Some remarks about concepts. *Brain and Behavioral Sciences, 1,* 557–560.

Brentano, F. (1960). The distinction between mental and physical phenomenon. In R. M. Chisholm (Ed.). *Realism and the background of phenomenology* (pp. 39–61). New York: Free Press.

Bretherton, I., & Beeghly, M. (1982). Talking about internal states: The acquisition of an explicit theory of mind. *Developmental Psychology, 6,* 906–921.

Bretherton, I., McNew, S., & Beeghly-Smith, M. (1981). Early person knowledge as expressed in gestural and verbal communication: When do infants acquire a "theory of mind"? In M.E. Lamb & L. R. Sherrod (Eds.). *Infant social cognition* (pp. 333–373). Hillsdale, NJ: Lawrence Erlbaum.

Broughton, J. (1978). Development of the concepts of self, mind, reality and knowledge. *New Directions for Child Development, 1,* 75–100.

Bruner, J. (1983). *Child's talk: Learning to use language.* Oxford: Oxford University Press.

Bruner, J. (1986). *Actual minds, possible worlds.* Cambridge, MA: Harvard University Press.

Byrne, R. W., & Whiten, A. (Eds.). (1988). *Machiavellian intelligence: Social expertise and the evolution of intellect in monkeys, apes, and humans.* Oxford: Oxford University Press.

Dennett, D. C. (1978). Beliefs about beliefs. *Brain and Behavioral Sciences, 1,* 568–570.

Dennett, D. C. (1987). *The intentional stance.* Cambridge, MA: MIT Press/Bradford Books.

Dunn, J. (1988). *The beginnings of social understanding*. Cambridge, MA: Harvard University Press.

Flavell, J. H. (1986). The development of children's knowledge about the appearance–reality distinction. *American Psychologist, 41,* 418–425.

Flavell, J. H., Everett, B. A., Croft, K., & Flavell, E. R. (1981). Young children's knowledge about visual perception: Further evidence for the Level 1–Level 2 distinction. *Developmental Psychology, 17,* 99–103.

Flavell, J. H., Flavell, E. R., & Green, F. L. (1987). Young children's knowledge about the apparent–real and pretend–real distinctions. *Developmental Psychology, 23,* 816–822.

Gopnik, A., & Astington, J. W. (1988). Children's understanding of representational change and its relation to the understanding of false belief and the appearance–reality distinction. *Child Development, 59,* 26–37.

Harman, G. (1978). Studying the chimpanzee's theory of mind. *Brain and Behavioral Sciences, 1,* 591.

Harris, P. (1989). *Children and emotion: The development of psychological understanding*. Oxford: Basil Blackwell.

Harris, P. L. (1990). The child's theory of mind and its cultural context. In G. Butterworth & P. E. Bryant (Eds.). *The causes of development* (pp. 215–237). London: Harvester Wheatsheaf.

Leekam, S. R. (1991). Jokes and lies: Children's understanding of intentional falsehood. In A. Whiten (Ed.). *Natural theories of mind: Evolution, development and simulation of everyday mindreading*. Oxford: Basil Blackwell.

Lempers, J. D., Flavell, E. R., & Flavell, J. H. (1977). The development in very young children of tacit knowledge concerning visual perception. *Genetic Psychology Monographs, 95,* 3–53.

Leslie, A. M. (1988). Some implications of pretense for mechanisms underlying the child's theory of mind. In J. W. Astington, P. L. Harris, & D. R. Olson (Eds.). *Developing theories of mind* (pp. 19–46). New York: Cambridge University Press.

Leslie, A. M. (1991). The theory of mind impairment in autism: Evidence for a modular mechanism of development. In A. Whiten (Ed.). *Natural theories of mind: Evolution, development and simulation of everyday mindreading* (pp. 63–78). Oxford: Basil Blackwell.

Lock, A. (Ed.). (1978). *Action, gesture and symbol: The emergence of language*. London: Academic Press.

Lock, A. (1980). *The guided reinvention of language*. London: Academic Press.

McCormick, P. (1990). *Quechua children's theory of mind*. Paper presented at the Sixth University of Waterloo Conference on Child Development, Waterloo, Ontario.

Mitchell, R. W., & Thompson, N. S. (Eds.). (1986). *Deception: Perspectives on human and non-human deceit*. Albany; State University of New York Press.

Moore, C., Pure, K., & Furrow, D. (1990). Children's understanding of the modal expression of speaker certainty and uncertainty and its relation to the development of a representational theory of mind. *Child Development, 61,* 722–730.

Moses, L. J., & Flavell, J. H. (1990). Inferring false beliefs from actions and reactions. *Child Development, 61,* 929–945.

O'Neill, D. K., Astington, J. W., & Flavell, J. H. (1992). Young children's understanding of the role that sensory experiences play in knowledge acquisition. *Child Development, 63,* 474–490.

Paley, V. G. (1981). *Wally's stories: Conversations in the kindergarten.* Cambridge, MA: Harvard University Press.

Paley, V. G. (1984). *Boys and girls: Superheroes in the doll corner.* Chicago, IL: Chicago University Press.

Perner, J., Leekam, S., & Wimmer, H. (1987). Three-year-olds' difficulty with false belief: The case for a conceptual deficit. *British Journal of Developmental Psychology, 5,* 125–137.

Peskin, J. (1992). Ruse and representation: On children's ability to conceal information. *Developmental Psychology, 28,* 84–89.

Piaget, J. (1928). *Judgment and reasoning in the child.* London: Kegan Paul. Originally published in French in 1924.

Pratt, C., & Bryant, P. E. (1990). Young children understand that looking leads to knowing (so long as they are looking into a single barrel). *Child Development, 61,* 973–982.

Premack, D., & Woodruff, G. (1978). Does the chimpanzee have a theory of mind? *The Behavioral and Brain Sciences, 1,* 515–526.

Ruffman, T. K., Olson, D. R., & Astington, J. W. (1991). Children's understanding of visual ambiguity. *British Journal of Developmental Psychology, 9,* 89–102.

Searle, J. R. (1969). *Speech acts: An essay in the philosophy of language.* New York: Cambridge University Press.

Shatz, M., Wellman, H. M., & Silber, S. (1983). The acquisition of mental verbs: A systematic investigation of the first reference to mental state. *Cognition, 14,* 301–321.

Stern, D. N. (1985). *The interpersonal world of the infant.* New York: Basic Books.

Wellman, H. M. (1985). The child's theory of mind: The development of conceptions of cognition. In S. R. Yussen (Ed.). *The growth of reflection in children* (pp. 169–206). San Diego, CA: Academic Press.

Wellman, H. M., & Bartsch, K. (1988). Young children's reasoning about beliefs. *Cognition, 30,* 239–277.

Wellman, H. W., & Estes, D. (1986). Early understanding of mental entities: A reexamination of childhood realism. *Child Development, 57,* 910–923.

Wellman, H., & Woolley, J. (1990). From simple desires to ordinary beliefs: The early development of everyday psychology. *Cognition, 35,* 245–275.

Wimmer, H., & Perner, J. (1983). Beliefs about beliefs: Representation and the constraining function of wrong beliefs in young children's understanding of deception. *Cognition, 13,* 103–128.

Yaniv, I., & Shatz, M. (1988). Children's understanding of perceptibility. In J. W. Astington, P. L. Harris, & D. R. Olson (Eds.). *Developing theories of mind* (pp. 93–108). New York: Cambridge University Press.

chapter 7

NARRATIVE COMPREHENSION
The Importance of Subjectivity
Lynne E. Hewitt

It is often difficult to relate theories of language, language learning, and language acquisition to specific challenges that arise in working with children. In this chapter, I describe how several purely theoretical ideas came together to suggest new directions in language therapy with an adolescent boy with autism. The chapter therefore has two purposes. The first is to illustrate an interactive approach to theory and practice. The second is to present an approach to narrative fiction that has been neglected in language therapy and education—that of considering narrative as an expression of subjective experience. All too often, the clinic and the academy are seen as somehow opposed in goals and in methods. In contrast, here I propose academic theory as the natural ally of clinical practice—two inseparable components of an organic process in our interaction with ideas and children.

NARRATIVE FICTION IN LANGUAGE THERAPY

The importance of narrative in language intervention has increased in recent years. One impetus behind this development has been the recognition that trying to teach language out of context is ineffective. Narratives offer a format to practice language use in extended discourse, and they have the advantage of being less open-ended and more structured than ordinary conversation. Speech-language pathologists who feel uncomfortable with the unconstrained nature of naturally occurring discourse may find narrative a comfortable compromise between traditional closed-ended language intervention and "just talking" (Culatta, 1984). A second factor in the rise of interest in narrative has been the recognition of a need to integrate language intervention with classroom goals. One type of narrative that figures prominently in language arts programs is fiction (Applebee, 1984; Brice-Heath, 1982). Brice-Heath (1982) argues that the ability to understand and interpret fictional texts according to the norms of the dominant culture is a crucial component of school success from the very earliest grades. The importance of fiction in education indicates a need for speech-language pathologists working with school-age children with language disorders to incorporate approaches to fictional language into their intervention plans.

Once the decision is made to incorporate fictional works into language therapy, the way clinicians think of narrative will affect which aspects they emphasize in their intervention. If narratives are thought of as a sequence of events unfolding in time, then plot-oriented analyses will be the primary focus. An example of such an approach is embodied in story-grammar analysis (Stein & Glenn, 1979), in which a normative schema of plot elements and their possible development is used to evaluate children's narratives. One way this approach has been used is to assess a child's ability to retell a story. Based on such an assessment, the clinician infers that deficits in comprehension arise from incomplete understanding of the story-grammar components. Intervention would then focus on teaching these elements (see, e.g., Carmin & Kind, 1985, and Gordon & Braun, 1983, cited in Scott, 1988).

Lahey (1988) outlines a different approach, focusing on two aspects of narrative structure: use of markers of narrative boundaries (such as "Once upon a time" and "The End") and adaptation to the listener, as evidenced by clear explanations and use of grammatical markers of narrative cohesion. The assessment of cohesive devices is based on Halliday and Hasan's (1976) work, in which they analyzed linguistic structures such as conjunctions and pronouns, producing a taxonomy of markers of cohesion. Their approach has been widely studied and used clinically to evaluate narrative competence in both adults and children (e.g., Liles, 1985).

In addition to the two types of analysis already described, Lahey also advocates use of Labov and Waletsky's (1967) approach to analyze narrative, in which a fundamental distinction is made between "evaluations" and narration and evaluative comments are seen as taking place off the "narrative line." Narration is the location of plot-related events; evaluations indicate the narrator's stance toward these events. Others have also advocated use of this approach to analyze children's fictional narrative (e.g., Bamberg & Damad-Frye, 1991). Because Labov and Waletsky developed their approach to analyze narratives of personal experience, and not for fictional narrative, some caution may be needed in using this method with fiction. Taking a functionalist perspective toward language entails that the structures observed in a given type of linguistic genre will be closely linked to the purpose of that genre. For example, Labov and Waletsky's finding that evaluative comments are important narrative structures may derive from an aspect of narration unique to oral communication. From this point of view, there is no reason to suppose that structures found appropriate to the analysis of one type of narrative will necessarily be appropriate for another.

Scott (1988), in her discussion of the types of analysis used to evaluate children's narratives, points out the importance of genre in evaluating children's narratives. She offers evidence that genre, context, and motivation all influence the nature of structures used by children. Scott argues that none of the narrative analyses thus far proposed is developed sufficiently to stand on its own as a means for teaching and evaluating narrative.

SUBJECTIVITY IN FICTION

In this chapter, I focus on the implications of taking an approach to fictional narrative in which the subjective nature of fiction is emphasized, along with its special nature as fiction. As narrative theorist Dorrit Cohn (1983) has observed, fiction is the only medium that offers us the illusion of directly experiencing the consciousness of another person. Another narrative theorist, Banfield (1982), argues that this aspect of fiction is its very essence, and that the language of modern narrative has evolved many unique structures purely to serve the purpose of fostering this illusion. Considered from this point of view, the fact that things happen in narratives—that they have plots—is secondary to the fact that individual experience, that is, subjectivity, is being represented.

The representation of experience in stories has also been called "perspective-taking." However this usage is ambiguous, since perspective-taking may occur in any form of discourse. For example, it might refer to the speaker's ability to take the listener's perspective for purposes of referencing in conversation. In this chapter, **perspective-taking** will be used in this broader sense, in which all discourse genres are included. In contrast, **subjectivity** will be reserved for the representation of consciousness in fiction. However, these two aspects of modeling of mental states are closely related.

The work of Jerome Bruner (1986) offers us a means for linking perspective in the broad sense and subjectivity in the narrow sense. He argues that the unique nature of narrative is due to its "dual landscape," in which there is a "landscape of action" (similar to traditional notions of plot and to story-grammar elements) and a "landscape of consciousness" (corresponding to what I have been calling subjectivity). Moreover, Bruner proposes that there exists a narrative mode of thought, distinct from the paradigmatic, logico-mathematical mode that predominates in the sciences. The narrative mode has received insufficient attention in psychology, according to Bruner. He suggests that this mode should be seen as at least equally important as the paradigmatic one as a means by which we understand the world. Bruner's argument suggests that subjectivity is pervasive in human thought and language. Evidence for this idea has also come from linguistics (Kuno, 1987). In this view, difficulty in comprehending subjective language and situations would result in difficulties in ordinary communication, and not just in comprehending fiction.

Evidence for the importance of subjective language in fiction has begun to accumulate. Wiebe (1990) expanded on Banfield's work, uncovering numerous linguistic devices for the representation of characters' psychological states, even in very simple literary works such as novels written for children. Wiebe's work suggests that subjective language pervades all aspects of fiction. Lucariello (1990) offers some experimental evidence for the importance of subjectivity as an organizing principle used by children in generating stories.

Using a Subjective Approach to Fiction

Talking about fiction in terms of subjectivity involves presenting stories as essentially a means for exploring the nature of people's lived experience. Analysis of fiction in terms of subjectivity involves examining the text for subjective contexts—places where the consciousness of one of the characters is being described or represented. Talking about the thoughts and feelings of characters leads naturally to a holistic approach to the text, that is, an approach in which plot elements, cohesive devices, and other elements of structure can naturally be seen to relate directly to the underlying purpose of representing individual experience.

Advantages of the Subjective Approach

All of the theories of narrative analysis previously outlined suggest means for evaluating children's comprehension and/or production of narrative in terms of an adult standard. The drawbacks of using adult models to evaluate children are well understood in other areas of language evaluation; one would not expect a normal young child to use adult syntax or phonology. In addition, use of any normative model will limit the clinician's ability to understand what the child him- or herself is doing. As in all areas of pragmatic language assessment and intervention, looking at the child's system on its own terms allows for the possibility of discovering systematicity and structure that is unique to the individual (Duchan, 1988; Lund & Duchan, 1993). The approach to narrative fiction to be proposed here, although admittedly drawn from adult models, is not normative; individual narrators are free to express the subjective experience of their characters by any means they can imagine.

Another way in which the subjective approach differs from other types of narrative analysis is that it alone addresses the issue of the goal of fiction. The other approaches discussed offer a taxonomy of components, but no explanation of what it means to engage in storytelling and story reading. An emphasis on subjectivity provides the child with an underlying purpose to the fictional narratives presented to him or her. This emphasis may be of particular benefit in facilitating comprehension because it focuses attention on reading and listening to stories as a form of lived experience, rather than merely as a task in which pattern and structure must be recognized.

USING THE SUBJECTIVE APPROACH TO NARRATIVE WITH LANGUAGE-DISORDERED CHILDREN

There is little research directly bearing on the ability of children with language disorders to comprehend and produce subjective elements in fiction. However, there is some evidence that subjectivity is likely to prove difficult for children with pragmatic language disorders. For one thing, facilitating comprehension of others' subjectivity acquires special significance if an explicit theoretical link is made between the ability to take another's perspective and the ability to communicate. An emphasis on subjectivity in therapy centered on narrative fiction will not only facilitate children's understanding of fiction, but may also help draw attention to the importance in all types of communication of putting oneself in another's place. In fact, one way of viewing pragmatic language disorders is as the linguistic manifestation of failing to take account of the listener's needs, implying an incomplete mental model of the listener's perspective. Such basic narrative skills as clarity in introducing and referring to different characters can be linked to the speaker's ability to take the point of view of the listener. There is evidence that these aspects of narrative are particularly difficult to master (Hemper, Picardi, & Tager-Flusberg, 1991; Peterson & Dodsworth, 1991). We may generalize the difficulty of perspective-taking in this broad, communicative sense to the specific case of representing different mental states in fiction. That is, if a clinician finds that a child has difficulty in providing the listener with clear references to characters, which involves taking the perspective of the listener, the child may well also have problems using language in the far more difficult task of expressing characters' subjective states. Receptively, he or she may have difficulty recognizing the linguistic markers of subjective contexts in fiction.

In what follows, I discuss the implications of the importance of subjective language in helping an individual with autism. There are theoretical reasons making subjectivity of particular interest in thinking about autism. But in emphasizing autism I do not mean to suggest that perspective-taking and the representation of consciousness in language are not important for all speakers. Quite the contrary is the case, in fact, given the growing body of evidence for the importance of this neglected area of language.

SUBJECTIVITY AND AUTISM

One population in which problems in pragmatic language use, as well as in understanding others, has been well documented is children with autism. "Autism" is a label that has been easier to apply than to define; it has proved difficult to find aspects of autism that are present in 100 percent of the individuals so labeled. However, at least two problem areas meeting this criterion have been identified: the presence of a pragmatic language disorder and difficulties in social interaction (Fay & Mermelstein, 1982; Tager-Flusberg, 1989). The exact relationship between these two areas has been the focus of debate. In recent years, a new model has been proposed, designed to offer a unified underlying basis for both social and linguistic deficits. According to proponents of this model, children with autism have a specific impairment in their ability to form mental models of others' mental states. Laboratory experiments designed to test children's ability to model others' beliefs have shown that children with autism consistently perform less well than mental and chronological age-matched controls (Baron-Cohen, 1989; Baron-Cohen, Leslie, & Frith, 1985, 1986; Leslie &: Frith, 1988; see also Astington, Chapter 6, for a review of research on this topic with typical children). Given that accurate mental models of others' beliefs are necessary for successful communication, several researchers (Baron-Cohen et al., 1985; Frith, 1989a, 1989b; Leslie, 1987; Tager-Flusberg, 1992) have proposed that these findings have uncovered the essential underlying basis for autistic people's linguistic and social difficulties. Although some (Boucher, 1989; Hobson, 1989, 1990) have questioned whether the "theory of mind" approach explains all problems associated with autism, it does help account for why pragmatics should give so much more difficulty than other areas of language. Moreover, it offers an intriguing basis for speculation regarding deficits in storytelling and story understanding in this population.

There are other, more indirect, sources of evidence suggesting, at minimum, that autistic people are aware of other people. Research indicates that children with autism behave differently with familiar and nonfamiliar caretakers (McHale, 1983), and that the social remoteness formerly cited as a hallmark of the syndrome, starting with its first describer, Kanner (1943), has been overstated (Mundy & Sigman, 1989). There is moreover much anecdotal

Although the results of this line of research do indicate that people with autism employ cognitive strategies that differ from those of typical individuals, the case for a special deficit in the ability to think about others' mental states has been undermined by two recent studies. These present evidence suggesting that children with autism are not devoid of comprehension of emotion. Yirmiya, Sigman, Kasari, and Mundy (1992) found that high-functioning children with autism performed much better than predicted on measures of empathy. In addition, Tager-Flusberg (1992) found that children with autism were comparable to Down syndrome controls in their spontaneous talk about desire, perception, and emotion.

evidence from those who know people with autism—the sense that people with autism, far from being remote and uninvolved, do try to communicate. The mere fact that verbal autistic individuals are able to engage in any sort of turn taking and topic maintenance in conversation suggests that they are aware that they are talking to someone. These findings offer the possibility that autistic people have some understanding of others, even if it is not fully and effortlessly expressed, as it is in typical individuals. Moreover, there is an ever-growing body of evidence coming out of those working with facilitated communication (Biklen, 1990; Makarushka, 1991) indicating that previous notions about the nature and scope of autism are seriously flawed.[1]

Despite the need for caution in interpreting the results of the theory of mind literature, those results cannot be ignored, particularly when considering to what degree people with autism are able to comprehend fiction. Astington (1990) explicitly links theory of mind models of child development and autism with Bruner's ideas about narrative, speculating that until children are able to make accurate models of other's beliefs, they will be unable to comprehend the representation of consciousness in fiction. And, one might add, given the critical importance of subjectivity in fiction, they will not be able to understand stories in any meaningful sense. Astington cites research by Baron-Cohen et al. (1986), finding that while autistic subjects were much better than mental age-matched controls at sequencing picture cards according to factors such as physical causation, they were much poorer than the controls at sequencing cards when inference about human motivation and state of mind was required. Even though picture cards are a far cry from real stories, this result provides some preliminary evidence for Astington's suggestions.

In an investigation comparing narrative storytelling in autism and Down syndrome, Loveland, McEvoy, Tunali, & Kelley (1990) found that the autistic subjects had greater difficulty retelling stories as a connected sequence of meaningful events. Other parameters such as recall of details did not differ between the two groups. The authors speculate that "a human cultural perspective seems to be lacking" from the narratives of autistic individuals. These authors do not discuss subjectivity as such; however, the language used to discuss their results is consistent with an interpretation suggesting that subjectivity was lacking from the narratives of the subjects with autism.

My own attention was first drawn to the link between subjectivity in narrative and the language of people with autism when I was shown an example of a narrative describing the movie *Splash* typed on a word processor by an autistic teenager I shall call "Dee."[2] Part of this narrative follows:

> I can see the boat, it's in the river. The boy and girl are going into the river and they're swimming under the water. . . .
>   The mermaid was taking a bath and her legs turned into a fish tail. Madison dried her legs. . . .
>   Allen and Madison are going to the debate. The man was hurting the

right arm and he got bandages on his right arm. The man was using the hose to spray Madison in New York City.

When she got wet, she got a tail. . . . The police took Madison to the big fish tank and put her in. The men in the white coats tested Madison and Allen. Madison was unhappy. Allen got her out of the big fish tank and into a car. The police chased them in water. Madison jumped into the water and she got into the fishy tail. The police were shooting at Allen and Madison. Allen jumped into the water and he was fighting with the divers. The divers was try to catch Madison. Allen and Madison won the fight. Allen and Madison kissed. They swam away and it was a happy ending.

I found two aspects of this narrative striking on first reading: the high level of accurate detail, combined with an overall feeling of somehow missing the point. None of the facts reported is incorrect. Yet this narrative contains only one explicit description of a psychological state (disregarding "it was a happy ending" as a formulaic ending with no reference to who was happy), and no language whose purpose is to depict the emotions of characters indirectly. Moreover, the one description of a subjective state in Dee's narrative is an extreme understatement: "Madison was unhappy." In fact, in this scene the character referred to is gravely ill and on the point of death. Earlier in Dee's manuscript (reproduced in the second paragraph), he describes a scene in which the mermaid is in the bath. Although the description is accurate, it omits the important fact that one character (Allen, not mentioned by Dee) is panicking while the other (Madison) is hurriedly trying to conceal something. In leaving out the characters' mental states he has left out the true meaning of events. In contrast, here is an oral description of the same scene produced by a normal adult:

> But anyway, once in a while while she's living with him she goes into the bathtub so she needs to join—get water once in a while. And when she's in the bathtub she turns into a mermaid. I mean her legs become fins again. And there's one episode where he comes home and she's in the bathroom, and she won't let him in, and she gets out of the tub and tries to dry herself, and he tries to break down the door, and he's worried about her.

This description captures many important psychological facts that Dee has omitted. And Dee is not only leaving out psychological descriptions. Plans and goals of the characters are not included in his version either, whereas they figure prominently in the narrative of the typical adult ("tries to break down the door"; "tries to dry herself"). The pervasive nature of human thoughts and emotions in narrative fiction, and the cost of leaving them out, becomes apparent when contrasting these two examples. To put Dee's narrative style in perspective, it is worth noting that in a study of the oral narratives of a five-year-old girl with typical to above-average language development, we found numerous examples of a wide variety of linguistic devices designed to convey subjectivity (Hewitt, 1992; Hewitt & Duchan, 1989). This child was able to manipulate various mental states, contrasting false beliefs and reality. She not only described mental states, but also depicted them indirectly with imaginative use of language. An example of part of one of her stories follows:

> So we just had to camp for a few days to get away from the worm.
> It was night and night and night, blew by, until finally appeared in his head what he could do.

In this example, the narrator achieves an almost poetic effect by mirroring the seeming endlessness of the night with lexical repetition; also note the vividness of the description of the character's thought as "appearing in his head." Even very young children can emphasize the psychological states of characters in ways that seem to elude Dee. Dee's writing is in some ways remarkably good, yet it lacks coherence because of its emphasis on isolated facts over the human motivations and emotions underlying the story.

One can look at Dee's narrative in two ways. It can be seen as evidence of a basic, irremediable deficit in comprehending other people, that is, as further support for the theory of autism claiming that autism is caused by a deficiency in the ability to model others' minds. Alternatively, one could view it less pessimistically, as offering a new perspective on what Dee needs to learn to improve his narrative. It may be that typical children learn that fiction is crucially about people and feelings without being explicitly taught. The fact that Dee does not seem to have learned this about fiction is not proof that he cannot learn it.

USING SUBJECTIVITY TO FACILITATE NARRATIVE COMPREHENSION IN A TEENAGER WITH AUTISM

Some years after seeing Dee's manuscript, I was asked to work with another teen-age boy with autism, whom I shall call Barry. Barry attends a typical high school with resource room support. He had successfully transferred to this environment following many years of placement in special schools. He had succeeded in math, science, history, and business courses, but he had not yet been enrolled in any English classes. These had been avoided out of concern that his language impairment would make English particularly difficult for him. One area that was considered a possible source of special difficulty for Barry was the emphasis on fiction in these courses. Since he could not graduate with a regular diploma without taking English and passing a state minimum competency test in it, the need to develop ability in this area was a priority.

In working with Barry, I chose to take an optimistic view of autistic people's understanding of others' minds. Rather than postulating that people with autism lack any "theory of mind," I hypothesized that they have a theory, but not the typical one. If one grants that some type of awareness of others' minds is not lacking in autism, then new directions for therapy are immediately suggested. That is, one may capitalize on whatever knowledge of mental states a person with autism does have, in order to help facilitate improved understanding of mental states in general. With this as my premise, I undertook to work with Barry on reading and discussing fictional narrative, with constant emphasis on comprehending and recalling the thoughts and feelings of the characters.

Prior to beginning therapy, I interviewed Barry to find out his ideas about stories and other forms of fiction such as movies and television.[3] When asked "Why do people tell stories?," Barry replied, "So they can (:) ge* a job (:) so they can learn about it and be a man." When asked "Can you tell me more?," Barry said, "And they tell stories so they can have good eyes." The first answer seems to imply some awareness of stories as a source of information. The second is difficult to interpret; further questioning did not elicit any explanation of what he meant. However, it seems to suggest some connection between reading and eyesight, as if reading were primarily a physical exercise.

I also elicited some simple narratives from Barry in order to determine what type of organization he would give to stories. In retelling familiar fairy tales, Barry left out numerous plot elements, as evidenced by the following recital of "Goldilocks and the Three Bears" (my backchannel remarks are omitted; B is Barry, L is Lynne):

B [The:] [Go* Goldi*] The three bears have a bowl of porridge and [the little girl] and a* Goldilocks ate the little bear's porridge. Three (:) bears were sitting in their chairs eating at the ca*, Goldilocks s* sat in the little bear's chair and Goldilocks slept in bed and Goldilocks was lying in the little bear's bed. And the little bear was sad.

L Ok, the little bear was sad and then what happened?

B [The*] Goldilocks ran away from the three bears. And got back and cried.

In this narrative Barry omits the patterning of events in which Goldilocks tries out each of the three bears' possessions in turn, finally settling on the baby bear's in each case. He omits mention of the three bears' point of view, as traditionally expressed through dialogue, instead using the generic (for Barry) adjective "sad" to convey the baby bear's distress at finding his possessions consumed, broken, and used without permission.

Analysis of Barry's retelling of "Little Red Riding Hood" provided support for the hypothesis that conceptualizing mental states was difficult for Barry. The text of Barry's retelling of "Red Riding Hood" follows:

B Little Red Riding Hood went (:) to her grandmother's house with some goodies in her basket and (:) the (:) wolf was hiding in her grandma's dre* bed. And (:) Goldilocks wore a red cape and a dress and she had* and the wood cutter

was cutting wood with an ax. And [five-second pause] and the* Goldilocks
ran away from the wolf.

L   Little Red Riding Hood, right? Yeah, um is that all?
B   Yep.
L   You don't remember any other parts to that story do you?
B   No.
L   What did Little Red Riding Hood think when she went into the room and the
    wolf was in her grandma's bed?
B   She was afraid.
L   Did she ever make a mistake in the story? Did she make a mistake?
B   Yup.
L   What?
B   (Gra*) The wolf sleeping in the grandma's bed.
L   What did she make the mistake about?
B   Don't know.

Barry mentions a psychological state when directly questioned, stating that
Little Red Riding Hood was afraid. He seems aware that there was something
peculiar about the wolf being in the grandmother's bed, as evidenced by
several false starts and mention of the fact in relation to any "mistake" made
by Little Red Riding Hood, but he is unable to articulate the crucial deception
aspect of the story.

Attempts to elicit plot summaries of books read in school were unsuccessful; Barry recalled few events and was not able to convey an idea of what
the books were about. This initial interview appeared to confirm the fears
expressed by his family, therapists, and teachers relative to his ability to handle
narrative fiction in a typical English class.

In working with Barry, I used a traditional lesson-style discourse format,
considering my task to be more like that of a teacher presenting new information than that of a therapist engaged in indirectly stimulating the development of new language forms. I used constant feedback on his answers to
questions about the texts read in order to make Barry aware of monitoring
characters' psychological states. A sample of a typical session follows:

L   Do you have any idea why she might have cried when her son said those bad
    things about himself?
B   Uh uh.
L   Why would that make a mother feel sad?
B   Itsa* It makes them afraid.
L   It makes him afraid? Umm, what about her feelings, what is she feeling?
B   Her feelings were hurt.
L   Um hm, I agree. How could her feelings have been hurt by him saying those
    things about himself?
B   I don't know. [almost inaudible]
L   OK, let's think about mothers. Today's Mother's Day, right? That's one reason
    I picked this story. How do mothers usually feel about their kids?
B   Sad.
L   All the time?
B   They feel happy.

L   Do they love them or hate them or they don't care?
B   They love them.

This excerpt shows the lesson-style format I chose for the process of drawing Barry's attention to the characters' feelings in the stories we read. In this early session, Barry had difficulty and tended to look for automatic responses that might relate to what I had asked. For example, I had asked what might make a mother feel sad, so when later asked how mothers usually felt about their children, Barry replied "sad." Given three choices, he was able to come up with a more conventional response with some confidence, showing an awareness of social norms in mothers' feelings for their children ("they love them"). Although this was a forced-choice task, the fact that Barry did not follow his usual tactic of repeating the last-offered choice suggests that he was consciously selecting his answer. Replies such as these provided evidence that Barry was able to reason about people's psychological states.

As therapy progressed, I found that Barry needed less explanation of events in the stories read, and he was better able to make inferences about characters' motivations and their impact on events in the stories. We primarily concentrated on reading a novel written for teenagers, *Light in the Forest,* by Conrad Richter. I selected this novel because its events turn almost entirely on the contrast among its various characters' belief systems. To help Barry understand this book, I continually focused his attention on the main character's thoughts and feelings. Barry had difficulty processing the multiple viewpoints in the book, and concentrating on one character's subjectivity seemed the best way to simplify the material for him.

Post-assessment was done several months following termination of therapy. I again requested Barry to talk about stories, to summarize a book he had read in school, and to tell again the two fairy tales he had told earlier. In questioning him about the novel read in English class, *Great Expectations* by Charles Dickens, I found he reported many psychological states: that Pip and Magwitch loved each other; that Estella was mean; that Pip and Estella fought; that Pip liked Miss Havisham. He had difficulty explaining the connection between Magwitch in the beginning of the book as the escaped convict aided by Pip and in the end as the rich man who has been Pip's anonymous benefactor for many years. In addition, Barry did not relate the story in a connected, chronological manner; his first attempt at plot summary was one sentence: "There's this boy Pip and he lives in England." Nonetheless, given the complexity and length (and archaic language) of this novel, Barry's grasp of essentials seemed fairly good.

Barry recalled several crucial psychological elements from the novel we read together in therapy. The plot of this novel involved a white boy captured by American Indians in infancy and forcibly separated from his adoptive Indian family, the only one he had ever known. Barry summarized this as follows: "There was an Indian in the forest and a boy. And the boy was mean. (Pause.) And the boy was nice. And he was weeping. (Lynne: Why?) Cause he couldn't find his mom and dad." The hesitation between "mean" and "nice" probably involves referencing problems. There is another character in the book, a young soldier who guards the captive and can fairly be described as "mean"; the main character is "nice." What is particularly striking here is the goal-oriented explanation of the reason for the boy's tears—he couldn't find his mother and father. These types of explanations were lacking in the initial interview and at the beginning of intervention.

In retelling "Goldilocks and the Three Bears," Barry this time included all plot essentials:

> Goldilocks. The three bears come to eat their porridge in a bowl in the kitchen and the porridge is cooking on the stove and it's steaming. And the three bears sit in their three chairs. And the three bears sleep in their three beds. And (:) the (:) three bears go out for a walk. And Goldilocks (:) was trying the hot porridge and it was too hot. And she was trying the middle sized bear's porridge and it's too cold and she tries the little bear's porridge and she ate it up! And (:) Goldilocks is sitting in the (:) great sized bear chair, and then the middle sized chair and then she's sitting in the little wee chair and the chair broke. Then Goldilocks is sleeping in the little wee bed and . . . (Lynne: Why did she pick that one?) Cause it was comfortable. The (:) bears come back for their porridge. And the little baby says someone's been eating my porridge and someone ate it all up. And the little wee bear said someone has broken my chair and has broken it all up. And the little wee bear said someone [unintelligible] slept in my bed and there she is. And Goldilocks [unintelligible] and she saw the bears and [unintelligible]. (Lynne: Yeah, they don't really say where she goes, do they?)

The impressive difference between versions 1 and 2 of "Goldilocks" is probably not primarily attributable to the intervention program that I designed. Barry started taking English after I began working with him, and this, in addition to the programs designed to help improve his language abilities by his school speech-language pathologist, and work with stories and writing in the resource room, had provided him with considerably more experience with stories by this time. Motivation may also have been a factor, although given the similarity of the pre- and postintervention interview formats, it is difficult to see why Barry's motivation to tell the story well should have changed so much. His retelling of "Little Red Riding Hood" differed little from the original one; he still failed to grasp that deception was involved, even under specific questioning:

L   But why did [the wolf] put on Grandma's clothes?
B   He looked funny.
L   Yeah, but why did he do it?
B   Cause Grandma ran away.
L   Did he want to look like Grandma?
B   No. (:)

L   Did Little Red Riding Hood make any mistake when she walked in—did she
    know right away that it was the wolf, or did she think it was her grandma?
B   It might* she thought it was a wolf! [heavy stress on "wolf"]

Barry's difficulty with this aspect of Little Red Riding Hood, coupled with
his difficulty understanding the dual nature of Magwitch in *Great Expectations*,
suggests that deception and dual identity are particularly difficult for him to
understand. It is interesting that this accords with the literature reporting
experiments designed to test autistic people's understanding of others' minds;
most of these tests involve deception of some sort.

Barry's ability to read and understand fiction still has a long way to go.
However, the intervention approach outlined here shows promise as one
means for facilitating Barry's comprehension of what he reads. Teaching him
to focus on the thoughts and feelings of characters offers him a tool for making
sense of what would otherwise be an unmotivated sequence of events. The
English classes he is taking do not require in-depth analyses of character or
interpretive essays. What they do require is recall of facts in the stories. If
Barry understands the stories as a whole—which, I have argued, involves
seeing them as representations of people's experiences—it will be much easier
to remember the details. Otherwise, he will have to memorize what amounts
to a list of unrelated events. In this sense, I see the intervention undertaken
with him as a means toward facilitating sense-making in stories.

CONCLUSION

In this chapter, I combined findings in two widely separated areas of research—narrative theory and the cognitive basis for autism—in order to develop an intervention program for a person confronted by some unusual
challenges, operating in an unusually supportive environment. But it is not
only the so-called "unusual" case that can benefit from a close marriage
between theory and practice; our day-to-day clinical work will always be
improved by incorporating specific ideas about how language works for those
who speak and understand it effortlessly. All the approaches to narrative
outlined in this chapter have their place, as long as each is used in accord
with its theoretical reason-for-being. In this sense, taking theory seriously
actually makes our work easier, because it gives us more ideas about how to
improve communicative competence in the children we treat.

NOTES

I am grateful to the Center for Cognitive Science at the State University of New York at Buffalo
for financial support which aided in the preparation of this chapter. In addition, I am grateful
to "Barry" and his family for their cooperation and assistance.

1. As yet there has been no published analysis of the pragmatics of the language expressed via facilitation; anecdotal accounts indicate that the language observed in this context may differ semantically and pragmatically from typical communication.
2. My thanks to Judith Duchan for showing me this example and first suggesting that it lacked subjective language.
3. Sessions with Barry were audiorecorded and transcribed. Transcription conventions are as follows: (:) indicates a pause; [] indicates transcriber's commentary; * indicates false starts and utterances broken off.

REFERENCES

Applebee, A. (1978). *The child's concept of story: Ages two to seventeen.* Chicago: University of Chicago Press.

Astington, J. (1990). Narrative and the child's theory of mind. In B. K. Britton & A. D. Pelligrini (Eds.). *Narrative thought and narrative language.* Hillsdale, NJ: Lawrence Erlbaum.

Bamberg, M., & Damrad-Frye, R. (1991). On the ability to provide evaluative comments: Further explorations of children's narrative competencies. *Journal of Child Language, 18,* 689–710.

Banfield, A. (1982). *Unspeakable sentences: Narration and representation in the language of fiction.* Boston: Routledge & Kegan Paul.

Baron-Cohen, S. (1989). Are autistic children "behaviorists"?: An examination of their mental–physical and appearance–reality distinctions. *Journal of Autism and Developmental Disorders, 19,* 579–600.

Baron-Cohen, S., Leslie, A., & Frith, U. (1985). Does the autistic child have a "theory of mind"? *Cognition, 21,* 37–46.

Baron-Cohen, S., Leslie, A., & Frith, U. (1986). Mechanical, behavioural and intentional understanding of picture stories in autistic children. *British Journal of Developmental Psychology, 4,* 113–125.

Biklen, D. (1990). Communication unbound: Autism and praxis. *Harvard Educational Review, 60,* 291–314.

Boucher, J. (1989). The theory of mind hypothesis of autism: Explanation, evidence, and assessment. *British Journal of Disorders of Communication, 24,* 181–198.

Brice-Heath, S. (1982). What no bedtime story means: Narrative skills at home and school. *Language in Society, 11,* 49–76.

Bruner, J. (1986). *Actual minds, possible worlds.* Cambridge, MA: Harvard University Press.

Cohn, D. (1983). *Transparent minds.* Princeton, NJ: Princeton University Press.

Culatta, B. (1984). A discourse-based approach to training grammatical rules. *Seminars in Speech and Language, 5,* 253–263.

Duchan, J. (1988). Assessment principles and procedures. In N. Lass, L. McReynolds, J. Northern, & D. Yoder (Eds.). *Handbook of speech-language pathology and audiology.* Philadelphia: B. C. Decker.

Fay, D., & Mermelstein, R. (1982). Language in infantile autism. In S. Rosenberg (Ed.). *Handbook of applied psycholinguistics: Major thrusts of research and theory* (pp. 393–428). Hillsdale, NJ: Lawrence Erlbaum.

Frith, U. (1989a). *Autism: Explaining the enigma.* Oxford: Blackwell.

Frith, U. (1989b). A new look at language and communication in autism. *British Journal of Disorders of Communication, 24,* 123–150.

Halliday, M., & Hasan, R. (1976). *Cohesion in English,* London: Longman.

Hemper, L., Picardi, N., & Tager-Flusberg, H. (1991). Narrative as an index of communicative competence in mildly mentally retarded children. *Applied Psycholinguistics, 12,* 263–279.

Hewitt, L. (1992). *Subjectivity in children's fictional narratives.* Unpublished manuscript, State University of New York at Buffalo, Department of Communicative Disorders & Sciences, Buffalo, NY.

Hewitt, L., & Duchan, J. (1989, April). *Subjectivity in child narratives: Beyond story grammars.* Paper presented at the meeting of the New York Speech-Language-Hearing Association, Kiamesha Lake, New York.

Hobson, R. P. (1989). Beyond cognition: A theory of autism. In G. Dawson (Ed.), *Autism: Nature, diagnosis, and treatment* (pp. 22–48). New York: Guilford Press.

Hobson, R. P. (1990). On acquiring knowledge about people and the capacity to pretend: Response to Leslie (1987). *Psychological Review, 97(1),* 114–121.

Kanner, L. (1943). Autistic disturbances of affective contact. *Nervous Child, 2,* 217–250.

Kuno, S. (1987). *Functional syntax.* Chicago: University of Chicago Press.

Labov, W., & Waletsky, J. (1967). Narrative analysis: Oral versions of person experience. In J. Helm (Ed.). *Essays on the verbal and visual arts.* Seattle: University of Washington Press.

Lahey, M. (1987). *Language disorders and language development.* New York: Macmillan.

Leslie, A. (1988). Pretence and representation: The origins of "theory of mind." *Psychological Review, 94,* 412–426.

Leslie, A., & Frith, U. (1988). Autistic children's understanding of seeing, knowing and believing. *British Journal of Developmental Psychology, 6,* 315–324.

Liles, B. (1985). Cohesion in the narratives of normal and language-disordered children. *Journal of Speech and Hearing Research, 28,* 123–133.

Loveland, K., McEvoy, R., Tunali, B., & Kelley, M. (1990). Narrative story telling in autism and Down's syndrome. *British Jounal of Developmental Psychology, 8,* 9–25.

Lucariello, J. (1990). Canonicality and consciousness in child narrative. In B. K. Britton & A. D. Pelligrini (Eds.). *Narrative thought and narrative language.* Hillsdale, NJ: Lawrence Erlbaum.

Lund, N., & Duchan, J. (1993). *Assessing children's language in naturalistic contexts.* (3rd ed.) Englewood Cliffs, NJ: Prentice Hall.

Makarushka, M. (1991, October 6). The words they can't say. *New York Times Magazine,* pp. 33–36, 70.

McHale, S. (1983). Social interactions of autistic and nonhandicapped children during free play. *American Journal of Orthopsychiatry, 53,* 81–91.

Mundy, P., & Sigman, M. (1989). Specifying the nature of the social impairment in autism. In G. Dawson (Ed.). *Autism: Nature, diagnosis, and treatment.* New York: Guilford Press.

Peterson, C., & Dodsworth, P. (1991). A longitudinal analysis of young children's cohesion and noun specification in narratives. *Journal of Child Language, 18,* 397–415.

Richter, C. (1990). *The light in the forest.* New York: Bantam Books.

Scott, C. M. (1988). A perspective on the evaluation of school children's narratives. *Language, Speech, and Hearing Services in Schools, 19,* 67–82.

Stein, N., & Glenn, C. (1979). An analysis of story comprehension in elementary school children. In R. O. Freedle (Ed.). *New directions in discourse comprehension* (Vol. 2). Norwood, NJ: Ablex.

Tager-Flusberg, H. (1989). A psycholinguistic perspective on language development in the autistic child. In G. Dawson (Ed.). *Autism: Nature, diagnosis, and treatment* (pp. 92–115). New York: Guilford Press.

Tager-Flusberg, H. (1992). Autistic children's talk about psychological states: Deficits in the early acquisition of a theory of mind. *Child Development, 63,* 161–172.

Wiebe, J. (1990). *Recognizing subjective sentences: A computational investigation of narrative text.* Doctoral dissertation, State University of New York at Buffalo, Department of Computer Science. (Tech. Rep. No. 90–03).

Yirmiya, N., Sigman, M., Kasari, C., & Mundy, P. (1992). Empathy and cognition in high-functioning children with autism. *Child Development, 63,* 150–160.

chapter 8

REPRESENTATIONAL PLAY AND STORY ENACTMENTS
Formats for Language Intervention
Barbara Culatta

Representational play and story enactments provide highly organized, motivating, and interactional contexts for facilitating and learning language. In play and story contexts the clinician guides the enactment of themes while implementing strategies to enhance a variety of linguistic goals. The approach permits the integration of content, form, and function; supports language by stimulating a child's a priori knowledge; and capitalizes on natural language learning processes. In this chapter, the rationale for using representational play and story enactments will be provided along with suggestions for implementing the approaches and incorporating strategies for achieving specific objectives.

It is within highly functional, interactive contexts such as those created during play and storytelling that children are motivated to associate meanings with their functions and forms (Brinton & Fujiki, 1989; Halliday, 1975; Wells, 1981, 1985, 1986). In such contexts, the selection of language rules is dictated by the speaker's need to specify content and achieve functions (Bloom & Lahey, 1978). Consider, for example, how the verb "to be" is exemplified when play participants negotiate roles. In representational play, children are invested in the roles they take and utterances such as "I be the doctor" serve to transform them into a desired character (Pellegrini & Galda, 1990).

In addition to integrating function, form, and content, scripted play and story contexts facilitate topically related turn taking. In scripted contexts, the child's participation in a conversational exchange is supported by the adult's guiding the exchange with devices that signal and prompt the child's response (Bruner, 1981 a & b, 1983; French, 1986; Lahey, 1988; Lucariello, Kyratzis, & Engel, 1986; Snow, 1984; Wells, 1981). In addition, the child's and adult's shared knowledge about the event, along with contextual information provided by props, serves to sustain topics across turns and utterances (Bloom, Rocissano, & Hood, 1976; Brinton & Fujiki, 1989; Lucariello et al., 1986; Nelson & Gruendel, 1979). The script provides predictablity that guides the exchange. For example, shared knowledge about grocery shopping and of the relationship that holds between the clerk and customer provides a supportive structure for maintaining a topically related exchange about where food items are located, how much they cost, and which products are better.

Just as play and story enactments can capitalize on script knowledge, they can also assist in elaborating that knowledge (Nelson, 1986; Nelson & Gruendel, 1981; Shugar & Kmita, 1990). Play and story enactment scenarios can provide a framework onto which new elements can be introduced (Nelson, 1986; Shugar & Kmita, 1990). In playing firefighters, the introduction of a ladder that is too short to reach a blaze can lead to novel attempts and outcomes and can permit the introduction of such elements as making sure the equipment is in working condition prior to responding to a call. Children's existing knowledge of firefighters using ladders and hoses to put out fires provides a framework onto which the new information can be related or associated (Nelson, 1986). Often that new information goes beyond the immediate, thus also facilitating the decontextualized use of language (Blank, 1983; Foster, 1986; French, 1986; Lucariello et al., 1986; Pellegrini & Galda, 1990).

Another advantage to play and story enactment approaches is that they blend linguistic with literacy goals by providing opportunities for the child to co-construct meaning from texts (Koppenhaver, Coleman, Kalman, & Yoder, 1991; and Yoder, 1992). Understanding the narrative voice, gaining meaning from print, and associating print with oral language can all grow out of play and story enactments (Koppenhaver et al., 1991, Pellegrini & Galda, 1990).

IMPLEMENTING THE REPRESENTATIONAL PLAY APPROACH

Representational play entails using props and assumed roles to recreate themes. The clinician must make decisions about how to support the development of the play scenario and maintain the interaction. In this approach the clinician decides about the theme or overall goal (get groceries, nurse a sick child, build a house); its subscripts or component events; and potential problems that could lead to new goals, attempts, and outcomes. Although making such decisions provides a framework for the clinician to follow, it does not mandate a rigid set of procedures. Encouraging the child to develop or at least co-construct the script is a crucial aspect of the approach (Shugar

& Kmita, 1990). An example of themes, component events, and potential problems appears in Table 8–1.

In the representational play approach, themes are selected on the basis of children's interests, script knowledge, and level of play development. According to Westby's (1988) developmental play scale, everyday activities (cleaning the house, taking care of baby, grocery shopping) and highly salient, memorable events (going to the doctor's, losing a pet) are the earliest play themes that children depict. Experienced events with modified outcomes (mom serving a chicken for dinner that isn't cooked) and observed events (playing police officer, firefighter, teacher) develop subsequently. The extent to which the theme and component events match the child's script knowledge determines the extent to which that knowledge will guide the child through the events (Nelson, 1986).

In addition to selecting themes and component events, the clinician also decides how to facilitate specific language and literacy goals within the play context. With individual children's needs and developmental levels in mind, decisions are made in the areas of narrative use, topically related turn taking, production of target forms and functions, decontextualized use of language, semantic knowledge, and literacy. A description of strategies that can be successfully embedded into a play context to achieve specific objectives follows.

Enhancing Narrative Skills

There is a close correspondence between play and narrative development, with play aiding and paralleling the development of narratives (Galda, 1984; Pellegrini & Galda, 1990). Play and narratives are structured in similar ways, with more advanced stages involving goals and plans and less advanced stages involving sequences of chronologically or causally related events (Pellegrini & Galda, 1990; Westby, 1988).

Narratives can be facilitated within the context of representational play in a variety of ways: by exemplifying specific narrative structures, by planning the play with the child, by guiding the play's development, and by supporting the child's contributions to the narrative structure.

Exemplifying narrative structures. Narrative development can be facilitated in play by providing the child with clear examples of select narrative structures. On the basis of the child's developmental level, the clinician can decide which narrative components to emphasize in play (i.e., temporally related events, causally related events, goal-directed behavior, or plans). For the child at the isolated scheme play level, temporally related events can be emphasized. For the child who produces action sequence narratives or engages in early multischeme combinatorial play, causal factors can be introduced in all-play contexts (flat tire on the way to the grocery store, hole in a shopping bag, cashier breaking a bottle). For the child who produces reactive sequence narratives or engages in evolving sequence play, with causal elements linking

TABLE 8-1 Themes and Component Events

DETERMINING THE EVENTS THAT COMPRISE A SCHEME/SCRIPT

Getting ready for school

Component events	Potential problems
getting dressed	can't wake children
brushing teeth	burn toast
waking children	can't locate shoes
packing lunches	dog runs away
locating assignments	car won't start
taking care of chores	child is sick
eating breakfast	Mom is in a bad mood

Traveling on an airplane

Component events	Potential problems
announce trip	child doesn't want to go
plan and pack	can't find ticket
load car	almost miss plane
drive to airport	attendant spills food
park car	baby gets sick
check in	set off alarm
go through security	plane develops problems
wait for plane	can't locate parachutes
board plane	plane crashes
fasten seat belts	
take off	
eat food	
land or crash	

Operating a store

Component events	Potential problems
set up store	put things in wrong places
describe product	can't locate product
locate product	find damaged merchandise
request information	can't find list
inspect products	break something,
	find unusual items
give money to cashier	give wrong amount in change
load purchases	get flat tire on way home

Running a school fair

Component events	Potential problems
decide purpose, plan	some rides are dangerous
make up games, rides	can't find parts, materials
decorate	food spills
make food	helpers don't come
set up rides, games	booths fall down
	rides don't work
children come to fair	children get lost, hurt, in trouble
children buy food	run out of hot dogs
conduct games	two children win, unfair rules

Learning to drive

Component events	Potential problems
learn parts of car	car has parts missing

TABLE 8–1 Themes and Component Events (cont.)

DETERMINING THE EVENTS THAT COMPRISE A SCHEME/SCRIPT

learn rules	rules don't make sense
start car	car has mechanical problems
drive	accidents happen, get lost, get stopped by police officer

Taking care of sick child

Component events	Potential problems
take temperature	
cover up baby	baby still cries
call doctor	doctor isn't available
dress warmly	
take to doctor	car won't start
hold baby while doctor examines	forget medicine
comfort baby	
take home	
give medicine	baby throws up medicine
give juice	mom falls asleep
put to bed	

Going to a restaurant

Component events	
Decide to go to restaurant	
get dressed	
call babysitter	
get baby ready	
drive to sitter	
give sitter instructions	
drive to restaurant	
Enter	
move self into restaurant	
wait to be seated	
follow to table	
sit down	
Order	
receive menu	
read menu	
decide what to order	spill drink
give order to waitress	
Eat	
waitress brings food	get wrong order
eat food	run out of food
ask for needed items	
comment on service	food is too hot
Exit	
ask for check	
give tip to waitress	
move to cashier	
pay for meal	
leave restaurant	
get baby from sitter	
drive home	

the events, goals and plans can be introduced (deciding ahead of time that the store worker will put things in the wrong places and the store owner will get angry). For children who are producing goals and plans, the clinician can guide the child's depiction of complex interrelated events.

Engage child in direct planning. A second way to enhance narrative knowledge is to engage the child in metalinguistic planning at the outset of the session. The clinician at first introduces the theme and characters (dolls and objects), solicits the child's agreement to participate, and permits the child to select a role.[1] Then, to the extent the child is capable, the clinician and child jointly make decisions about the goals, plans, attempts, and outcomes. For children who are not yet capable of joint planning, the clinician gives the child suggestions or choices for initiating events, goals, outcomes, and characters' reactions. If unable to engage the child's participation, the clinician states the goal (Let's pretend Mom and Dad get a babysitter and go out for dinner) and solicits the child's agreement (Want to pretend the babysitter doesn't do a good job taking care of the baby?). Even with children who are at an evolving schematic play level, some level of planning is generally modeled (e.g., in creating a birthday party for Bert, Ernie, need to plan whom to invite, what to serve, what presents to buy or make, and how to decorate the room).

Guiding the development of the narrative. In addition to planning at the outset, the clinician can adopt various narrative modes or voices to impose an organized narrative framework onto the play as it develops (Pellegrini & Galda, 1990; Wolf & Hicks, 1989). The use of different voices (stage manager, character, narrator) provides the play with a structure that is layered rather than sequential, with the layers conforming to various levels of a narrative (Pellegrini & Galda, 1990). These layers are reflected in the voices the players use in directing and participating in the play (Pellegrini & Galda, 1990; Westby, 1988; Wolf & Hicks, 1989). When adopting the narrator voice, the player functions as an observer, relating the main theme and commenting on the events and story structure elements as they evolve (e.g., "The babysitter doesn't look like she really wants to watch your baby"). When adopting the character's voice, the player talks from the perspective of a participant in the event and says what the character would say (e.g., "I couldn't find the baby's medicine"). When adopting the stage manager voice, the participant steps out of the play to plan its development, negotiate the conduct of the participants, and guide the play to a logical conclusion (e.g., "Let's pretend that the babysitter falls asleep and can't find the baby when she wakes up"). Although the stage manager voice is the one that most obviously contributes to the planning because of its metalinguistic nature, all three voices aid in the organization of the story. In the stage manager voice the clinician provides direct comments about the play, whereas in the character and narrator roles the clinician provides the feelings, assumptions, and intents that frame the play's development.

Supporting the child's contributions.   The clinician not only adopts the use of all three voices to guide the play, but also responds to the contributions the child makes in each voice. All contributions that the child makes to the script are incorporated into the play unless they become too repetitive (e.g., child **only** wants to take care of babies), violate script knowledge (e.g., wants to leave the restaurant without paying, unless not paying is a planned event), or impinge on the rights or feelings of the other characters (e.g., insists that another character **must** order pizza). For example, in a "Christmas Shopping at a Mall" script, one child wanted to leave the shopping center without the other characters. The clinician, using the stage manager voice, insisted that she did not have the right to leave without consulting the other characters. A negotiated agreement resulted.

Facilitating Topically Related Turn Taking

During the course of the play, the clinician enhances topically related turn taking by providing goals, making assertions, contriving reasons to communicate, signaling the child's turn, and responding to the child's initiations.

Providing goals.   Ongoing topically related turn taking exchanges are maintained by having the child and clinician encounter reasons for interacting. These reasons are dictated, in part, by the overall theme or goal of the play. Collaborating to surprise Ernie with a birthday party and needing to work together to put out fires are examples of events that necessitate ongoing turn taking and collaboration. These ongoing reasons for interacting can take the form of obstacles, problems, or complications that interfere with overall goal attainment (see Table 8–1). As the characters attempt to solve problems that are interfering with ultimate goal attainment, reasons for collaborating are found (Shugar & Kmita, 1990).

Making assertions.   Reasons for interacting are also incorporated into the play when informational assertions are made by the clinician. The assertions take the form of expressions of feelings, directions, and statements appropriate to the story line (e.g., I want to decorate for the party all by myself. I'm not sure where we can put all this stuff. That man won't let me bring my dog into the store). Expressions of feelings between participants motivate a variety of conversational functions (Dore, 1986), while directions and statements made by the clinician's character constrain the child's responses (Shugar & Kmita, 1990). The information supplied by the clinician serves as a structuring device to guide the discourse (Shugar & Kmita, 1990).

Contriving reasons to communicate.   In addition to providing underlying content for maintaining topically related turn taking, certain clinical devices serve to increase the likelihood that the child will initiate or extend current topics. Strategies that pass the turn back to the child and increase the likelihood that the child will initiate abound in the literature (Brinton & Fujiki, 1989; Culatta, 1984; Fey, 1986; Lucas, 1980). These include:

1. *Requiring the child to convey information.* By increasing the number of characters (stuffed or real), the clinician increases the opportunities for information to be conveyed. For example, in acting out a birthday party, information needs to be conveyed to the guests about what type of party, what to bring, and how to assist in planning. In a grocery store, the child, as clerk, must provide directions to helpers, assist customers in locating merchandise, and describe new products.

2. *Requesting information.* In this strategy the clinician, as one of the characters, needs information in order to achieve a goal. As a cook's helper, the clinician could state, "I don't know how to make this" or "How does this toaster work?"

3. *Violating usual occurrences.* In this strategy the clinician arranges for the child to encounter unusual events or violations of routines. Handing the child the wrong item and having needed objects altered or missing are examples.

4. *Providing the child with choices and decisions to make.* In this strategy the clinician provides the child with choices relative to the conduct of the play. As a waitress, the clinician can ask her boss, "Do you want me to clean up the dining room or wait on customers?"

5. *Providing inaccurate information.* Presenting the child with inaccurate information can elicit the child's refutation. In the context of cleaning a house, the clinician can insist that the broom won't work or that a very dirty wall is clean.

Signaling turn allocation. Strategies for passing the turn back to the child consist of silence, proximity, and gaze (Brinton & Fujiki, 1989). To increase the likelihood that the child will fill his or her turn, the clinician focuses attention on the child and waits expectantly for a response.

Responding to the child's initiations. The clinician can facilitate topically related turn taking by being responsive to the child's initiations (Shugar & Kmita, 1990). The clinician can acknowledge and comment on the child's actions and can repeat and elaborate the child's utterances. In these ways the clinician builds a "topical framework" around the child's contributions (Brinton & Fujiki, 1989).

Facilitating Decontextualized Language Use

Decontextualization, the ability to use language to represent events removed in time and space, is an important linguistic attainment that can be facilitated within the play context (Blank & Marquis, 1987; Blank, Rose, & Berlin, 1978; Dickinson, 1990a, 1990b). Decontextualized language can be introduced by selecting abstract props and by making references to remote events.

Abstractness of props. Westby (1988) provides a developmental guideline for prop selection on a contextualized to decontextualized continuum:

from real objects to replicas, object transformations (using a box as a garage), construction toys (blocks become telephones and roads are created with sand) and no props at all (language alone is used to set scenes and roles). The extent to which props are used depends on the child's capacity to move beyond the props to set scenes, situations, and roles. For all children there will be some blending of contextualized and decontextualized prop use. When real objects serve as the primary type of representation, the clinician also introduces absent objects and object transformations (e.g., real food containers and pretend absent money used within the same grocery store scenario). Even when language is the primary mode of representation, some real objects are used to motivate and guide the play's development (e.g., the presence of paper vs. plastic bags in a grocery scene can trigger a discussion of which is better) (Pellegrini & Galda, 1990).

Referring to remote events. Decontextualization also occurs by having the clinician discuss, explain, and predict events that are removed in time and space. In a grocery store context, the clinician can explain why certain foods are weighed and why people can't eat the food until it is paid for. One child didn't know how stores got their food or that the workers got paid, or that the "owner" was the one who got to be the ultimate boss. Discussing events that are beyond the immediate play context and then illustrating them (e.g., pretending to go to the food distributor to get food and having the "owner" pay his or her helpers for specific work) are means for helping the child move from immediate decontextualized language use (Blank, 1990; Dickinson, 1990a, 1990b). Discussing the play at the end of the session, relating it to parents, writing the play as a story, and talking about how the play relates to events in the child's life are additional ways to expose the child to decontextualized language.

Enhancing the Expression of Communicative Functions

Throughout the play the clinician has the opportunity to repeatedly model conversational functions and to arrange for the child to need to convey a variety of functions. The clinician expresses functions by negotiating roles and plans; projecting events; stating rules, goals, and assumptions; and expressing the feelings, needs, desires, and intentions of the characters. Children who tend to be overly assertive are likely to become more responsive when the clinician patiently explains his or her own perspective or the perspective of the characters (through character dialogue, stage manager voice, or narrator). Children who tend to be overly passive, or who fail to exhibit particular functions, can encounter contrived reasons to express certain functions. For example, a child who is not using language to seek information can be provided with insufficient information (e.g., "You make cookies by putting the ingredients in a bowl"), the need to obtain information (e.g., "I need to know how this works, can you ask the store owner?"), or unspecified referents (e.g., saying "you can take that with you" without the object referred to being present or obvious).

Training Syntactic Form

To facilitate the development of grammatical structures, the clinician determines ahead of time the overall complexity of input he or she will use and any particular grammatical forms to be targeted. Once the structural objectives have been set, the clinician models selected targets and provides the child with opportunities to use those targets.

Modeling target structures. Representational play permits the modeling of target forms in contexts that exemplify their meaning and function. Modeling makes the correct form salient and serves to remind the child to use it. Within the play context, the clinician arranges to frequently need to convey functions that require target structures (Culatta, 1984; Culatta & Horn, 1982; Kirchner, 1991). For example, searching for missing clothes increases the likelihood of expressing the copula in such utterances as "Here is my sock. Now, where is my shoe? My shoe is lost. I can't find my shoe. My shoe is not here." Or, providing alternatives during dressing can require the expanded noun phrase (e.g., "I want to wear this fancy blue shirt" or "This plain brown jacket makes me look like Daddy"). More structured, repetitive play sequences can be selected when targets are first being introduced and when it is necessary to highlight the target for a child who is not producing it at acceptable levels (Brinton & Fujiki, 1989).

Opportunity to use target forms. For children with expressive language difficulty (restricted language forms), opportunities to use targets can be incorporated into the play. During a "taking girl scouts to an amusement park" theme, the clinician evoked the future modal "will" by problem solving (We can't find Susan, what will we do?), arranging for the girls to make plans (I will go to the Merry-Go-Round, what will you do?), and predicting which girls will go where (e.g., Mary will go on the ferris wheel), and in planning (e.g., She will meet us at the snack shop). A store theme can provide the child with opportunities to produce questions in the role of clerk or customer. If the child fails to use an obligated target, the clinician expands the child's production and provides imitative support (Culatta, 1984; Culatta and Page, 1982; Culatta & Horn, 1982).

Enhancing semantic knowledge and use

Within any play context, the clinician is provided with opportunities to enhance semantic knowledge by highlighting relevant lexical-referential connections and by using language the child already knows to describe or define new words. Decisions regarding which words to teach are made on the basis of the child's existing knowledge and the content of the theme. Words incidental to the script (e.g., words such as *rinse, sudsy, customer,* and *appointment* in a beauty parlor theme) and words that are not content specific (e.g., words such as *each, next to, still, full, kind of,* and *supposed to*) are selected as targets. For one child, Amy, the words *rinse, cooperate* (be patient), *knotty, customer, waiting area,* and *supplies* were selected as objectives specific to a beauty parlor scenario while the terms *prepare, still,* and *supposed to* were among targets incorporated into many themes. For a developmentally younger child, Allison, the scenario specific words selected were *rinse, soapy,* and *pour* while the more general targets included *wait, use, need,* and *get.* In both cases, the clinician used gestures, multiple exaggerated examples, and recastings to highlight the words (e.g., These are the supplies. These are the things we will need to use. We can line up the things we need. We need shampoo and conditioner and scissors. These are our supplies, the things we need).

Enhancing Literacy

Opportunities to gain meaning from written text can be embedded into the scripted play contexts. The clinician can assist the child in writing and revising the enacted scenarios and then sharing those written stories with others. Other techniques for giving meaning to print and for incorporating print into the play context include labeling items and settings (e.g., "store," "yard sale," and "snack shop"), sorting items according to their labels (meat vs. produce), making lists, writing notes, and conveying written messages and directions to the characters.

In summary, representational play provides a facilitative context for the acquisition of a variety of linguistic skills. The facilitative context, along with intervention strategies that are incorporated into it, serves to enhance the attainment of multiple integrated goals. All of the objective areas discussed (topically related turn taking, production of narratives, semantic knowledge, production of forms and functions, decontextualized use of language, and literacy) overlap. For example, the process of having characters divide chores necessitates the negotiating function, uses language in a decontextualized way, and exemplifies vocabulary such as *fair, supposed to, chore,* and *lazy.* Likewise, the use of the stage manager voice serves to promote the development of the narratives, provides opportunities to use language in decontextualized ways, and models specific content, forms, and functions.

IMPLEMENTING THE STORY ENACTMENT APPROACH

Story enactment differs from the representational play only in that the events represented are depicted in texts. Story enactments, because they are based in written stories, provide additional opportunities for facilitating literacy and narrative skills. Literacy skills are facilitated because the text is an integral part of the exchange and because story retellings and enactments improve comprehension (French, 1988). Narrative skills are facilitated because the child is systematically exposed to texts that represent explicit narrative structures such as action sequences, reactive sequences, or episodes.

Selecting Texts

Prior to implementing the story enactment approach, the clinician selects appropriate text materials. Books are selected on the basis of the child's world knowledge, interests, and level of linguistic or conceptual development. Books with predictable and repetitive elements, which are often simple action sequences, are useful for children who are at an early narrative level, who have deficits in form, or who need tightly framed events to support turn taking (Kirchner, 1991). Kirchner argues that the fixed phrases that appear in predictable, repetitive texts can provide a foundation from which subsequent linguistic analyses can take place. Once productions are fairly well learned, they can be varied by rephrasing, expanding, and substituting. Kirchner holds that controlled variation along with frequent exposure to particular language forms permits children to learn linguistic patterns as well as their functions in discourse.

Action sequences that consist of events chronologically linked are useful for children who are not yet connecting elements in play or language. Reactive sequences, which contain chains of causally related events and simple episodes, are appropriate for children whose narratives and play consist of action sequences or evolving schematic representations. Texts with simple but highly discernible story structure elements should be considered for children whose play or story-telling lack causality, planning, or goal directedness (i.e., whose play and narratives consist of simple action sequences or evolving schematic representations). If the child exhibits some narrative elements (goals, attempts, and consequences), texts with planning should be emphasized so that the child can be exposed to how characters' thoughts and plans affect attempts and outcomes.

Reading and Acting Out the Stories

Selected stories are introduced with a simple overview. The clinician then reads or tells the story while adjusting the complexity of structure and content and amount of detail to the child's conceptual and linguistic levels. To work on comprehension during the reading/telling process, the clinician focuses the child's attention on major story components, commenting on critical elements, drawing parallels between the text and the child's experiences, and using intonation and gestures to illustrate meanings. Commenting on elements that go beyond the text not only activates the child's understanding but also helps the child to move from contextualized to decontextualized language. The clinician should be careful, however, to focus comments on critical story grammar components rather than on irrelevant details.

Once the clinician has read the text, he or she can reread it using intonation and the cloze procedure, pausing at critical junctures, to engage the child's participation (Kirchner, 1991). Depending on the child's motivation, stories can be read a number of times to develop familiarity, word recognition, and fluency.

The clinician and child then assume roles and act out the story with props. This is done with the clinician making direct references to the text and making explicit correspondences between printed and spoken words as he or she narrates the story. During the enactment, focus is once again placed on major story grammar components—initiating events, reactions, goals, plans, and consequences. The story may be reenacted several times, depending upon the child's interest, altering props, alternating roles, and gradually reducing supports until the child is assuming most of the responsibility for telling. Letting the child act as the "announcer" or narrator, telling the story with paper cut-out props, telling the story to peers or into a recorder, and rewriting the story are also strategies for providing additional opportunities to retell and to associate text with meaning.

Achieving Specific Objectives

The same strategies for achieving specific objectives and language facilitation techniques that were outlined in the representational play approach apply to story enactments. During book reading and story enactments, the clinician can explain the meaning of new words, adjust complexity of input, model target forms, exemplify meanings nonverbally (through gestures, exaggerated actions), and provide opportunities to use targets.

SUMMARY

This chapter has outlined various ways in which representational play and story enactment can be used to facilitate language learning in children. It was shown how play contexts can be structured to provide children with opportunities for learning narrative structuring, turn taking, decontextualized language use, language form and function, and literacy skills. It was also shown how clinicians can use stories to help children learn language. Through careful selection and presentation of stories, and by providing support for the children to act the stories out, clinicians can create situations which are motivating and accessible to children with language-learning problems.

NOTE

1. Although the child is given the opportunity to select his or her desired role, role reversal is expected, with explanations often given that it is only fair that both or all participants get a chance to play all roles. By incorporating role reversal into the play scenario, the clinician is assured of the opportunity to elaborate sequences and to demonstrate various conversational functions and forms.

REFERENCES

Blank, M. (1983). *Teaching learning in the preschool: A dialogue approach.* Cambridge, MA: Brookline Books.

Blank M. (1990, March). *The language of discourse.* Workshop presented at Bradley Hospital, Providence, Rhode Island.

Blank, M., & Marquis, M. A. (1987). *Directing discourse: Eighty situations for teaching meaningful conversation to children.* Tuscon, AZ: Communication Skill Builders.

Blank M., Rose S., & Berlin, L. (1978). *The language of learning: The preschool years.* New York: Grune & Stratton.

Bloom, L. & Lahey, M. (1978). *Language Development and Language Disorders.* New York: Wiley.

Bloom, L., Rocissano, L., & Hood, L. (1976). Adult–child discourse: Developmental interaction between information processing and linguistic knowledge. *Cognitive Psychology, 8,* 521–522.

Brinton, B., & Fujiki, M. (1989). *Conversational management with language-impaired children.* Rockville, MD: Aspen.

Bruner, J. S. (1981a). The social context of language acquisition. *Language and Communication, 1,* 155–178.

Bruner, J. S. (1981b). The pragmatics of acquisition. In W. Deutsch (Ed.), *The child's construction of language* (pp. 39–57). London: Academic Press.

Bruner, J. S. (1983). *Child's talk: Learning to use language.* New York: W. W. Norton & Co.

Culatta, B. (1984). A discourse based approach to training grammatical rules. *Seminars in Speech and Language, 5,* 253–263.

Culatta, B., & Horn, D. (1982). A program for achieving generalization of grammatical rules to spontaneous discourse. *Journal of Speech and Hearing Disorders, 47,* 174–180.

Culatta, B., & Page, J. (1982). Strategies for achieving generalization of grammatical constructions. *Communicative Disorders, 7,* 31–44.

Dickinson, D. (1990a). Review of relevant research: Long-term effects of facilitating oral language development. In E. Tittnich, L. Bloom, R. Schomburg, & S. Szekers (Eds.), *Facilitating children's language: Handbook for child related professionals* (pp. 35–57). Binghamton, NY: The Haworth Press.

Dickinson, D. (1990b). Implications for organizing an appropriate language program. In E. Tittnich, L. Bloom, R. Schomburg, & S. Szekers (Eds.), *Facilitating children's language: Handbook for child related professionals* (pp. 59–65). Binghamton, NY: The Haworth Press.

Dore, J. (1986). The development of conversational competence. In R. L. Schiefelbusch (Ed.), *Language competence: Assessment and intervention.* San Diego, CA: College-Hill Press.

Fey, M. (1986). *Language Intervention with young children.* San Diego, CA: College-Hill Press.

Foster, S. (1986). Learning discourse topic management in the preschool years. *Journal of Child Language, 13,* 231–250.

French, L. (1986). The language of events. In K. Nelson (Ed.), *Event knowledge: Structure and function in development.* Hillsdale, NJ: Lawrence Erlbaum.

French, L. (1988). Story retelling for assessment and instruction. *Perspectives for Teachers of the Hearing Impaired, 7* (2), 20–22.

Galda, L. (1984). Narrative competence: Play, story telling, and comprehension. In A. Pellegrini & T. Yawkey (Eds.), *The development of oral and written language in social context* (pp. 105–119). Norwood, NJ: Ablex.

Halliday, M. A. K. (1975). *Learning how to mean: Explorations in the development of language.* London: Edward Arnold.

Kirchner, D. (1991). Reciprocal book reading: A discourse-based intervention strategy for the child with atypical language development. In Gallagher, T. (Ed.), *Pragmatics of language: Clinical practice issues.* pp. 307–332. San Diego, CA: Singular Publishing Group.

Koppenhaver, D. A., Coleman, P. P., Kalman, S. L., & Yoder, D. E. (1991). The implications of emergent literacy research for children with developmental disabilities. *American Journal of Speech Language Pathology, 1,* 38–44.

Lahey, M. (1988). *Language disorders and language development.* New York: Macmillan.

Lucas, E. (1980). A remediation procedure for language disorders. In E. Lucas, *Semantic and pragmatic language disorders* (pp. 197–221). Rockville, MD: Aspen.

Lucariello, J., Kyratzis, A., & Engel, S. (1986). Event representations, context, and language. In K. Nelson, (Ed.), *Event knowledge: Structure and function in development.* Hillsdale, NJ: Lawrence Erlbaum.

Nelson, K. (1986). Event knowledge and cognitive development. In K. Nelson (Ed.), *Event knowledge: Structure and function in development.* Hillsdale, NJ: Lawrence Erlbaum.

Nelson, K. & Gruendel, J. M. (1979). At morning it's lunchtime: A scriptal view of children's dialogues. *Discourse Processes, 2,* 73–94.

Nelson, K., & Gruendel, J. (1981). Generalized event representations: Basic building blocks of cognitive development. In M. E. Lamb & A. L. Brown (Eds.), *Advances in developmental psychology* (Vol. 1, pp. 131–158). Hillsdale, NJ: Erlbaum.

Pellegrini, A. D., & Galda, L. (1990). Children's play, language and early literacy. *Topics in Language Disorders, 10* (3), 76–88.

Shugar, G. W., & Kmita, G. (1990). The pragmatics of collaboration: Participant structure and the structures of participation. In G. Conti-Ramsden & C. Snow (Eds.), *Children's language* (Vol. 7, pp. 273–303). Hillsdale, NJ: Lawrence Erlbaum.

Snow, C. (1984). Parent–child interaction and the development of communication ability. In R. L. Schiefelbusch & J. Pickar (Eds.), *The acquisition of communicative competence* (pp. 69–108). Baltimore, MD: University Park Press.

Wells, G. (1981). *Learning through interaction.* New York: Cambridge University Press.

Wells, G. (1985). *Language development in preschool years.* New York: Cambridge University Press.

Wells, G., (1986). *The meaning makers.* Portsmouth, NH: Heinemann.

Westby, C. (1988). Children's play: Reflections of social competence. *Seminars in Speech and Language, 9* (1), 1–14.

Wolf, D., & Hicks, D. (1989). The voices within narratives: The development of intertextuality in young children's stories. *Discourse Processes, 12,* 329–351.

Yoder, D. (1992, April). *Literacy and children with speech and physical impairments.* Seminar presented at the University of Rhode Island, Kingston, Rhode Island.

chapter 9

CHILDREN'S DEVELOPMENT OF SCRIPTAL KNOWLEDGE

Gail S. Goodman, Judith Felson Duchan,
and Rae M. Sonnenmeier

Research has shown that children's abstract knowledge of familiar everyday events strongly influences their ability to engage in social interaction during those events, to express themselves verbally as they participate in them, to remember the relevant and idiosyncratic particulars of the events at a later time, and to describe the relevant aspects of those events to someone else (Bruner, 1983; Farrar & Goodman, 1992; Nelson & Gruendel, 1981). Thus the study of what children know about everyday events is necessary for understanding language acquisition in typical and atypical learners, and it is crucial for developing sensitive assessment and intervention approaches for facilitating language in children diagnosed as language disordered.

In this chapter we present what has been learned about the structure of mental representations of events and how they are used by children and adults. We describe some of the factors that affect the use of event representations in specific situations and propose a theoretical model for how children typically learn event representations. Finally, we provide support for the model from a series of studies that have examined typical children's script formation and use in remembering events.

HOW EVENT REPRESENTATIONS ARE STRUCTURED AND WHAT THEY INCLUDE

Children's knowledge of events has been studied under the aegis of schema theory (Mandler, 1984; Nelson, 1986; Rumelhart, 1980). A **schema** is an organized cognitive structure; that is, an organized mental representation of knowledge about some entity, be it an object, a scene, or an entire event (Mandler, 1979). This representation is formed based on an individual's experience with the entity. It consists of expectations for what things in the world look like or how they ordinarily behave (Mandler, 1979). Schemas are thought to be hierarchically organized, with specific parts subsumed by more general information (Nelson, 1986). For example, a schema for a nose is embedded in a schema for a face which is embedded in a schema for a body. From early childhood, schemas form an important part of an individual's knowledge base; in fact, they have been considered by some to be the earliest form of cognitive organization in children (Nelson, 1986).

Schemas assist individuals in making sense out of the world around them (Lund & Duchan, 1993). Bartlett (1932) proposed that individuals use schemas to remember or reconstruct objects or events, using old information to interpret new information. Since certain expectations are associated with a schema, recalling a fragment can lead to activation of the whole schema. This makes cognitive processing more economical.

Besides providing a way to recognize and predict the occurrence of objects or events, schemas help individuals identify novel aspects of events. The fact that children and adults can recall the autobiographical particulars as well as the general characteristics of events lends support to a distinction between "episodic" representations—that include specific details of particular personally experienced events—and "generalized event representations" that include general features of grouped events. (Nelson, 1986; Tulving, 1972). One can remember last night's dinner as a specific event: that an argument took place, that the water spilled, and that the baby asked for more milk for the first time; one can also remember meals in general, that is, typical meals at home with participants sitting at designated places and interacting in usual ways.

A **script** is a type of schema. The term *script* is usually reserved for representations of regularly occurring activities that have been routinized. Our knowledge of events such as going to the dentist, going to a birthday party, or cooking dinner is of events organized into well-learned scripts.

Schank and Abelson (1977) first defined a script as a mental representation of an ordered sequence of actions related to a particular context, including the spatial and temporal information relevant to the context. A script is also organized around a social goal. The actors, actions, and objects used to carry out those goals are specified. Scripts contain slots and requirements about what can fill those slots. A script, like other schema types, contains certain defaults that are assumed if the person, action, or object is not specified. That is, people fill in the items based on their knowledge of a general script for an event even if the items are not explicitly mentioned. Also, like other schemas, scripts are general structures used in the processing of particular events. Unlike many other schemas, scripts involve actions as well as temporal and causal relations between the actions.

Nelson and her colleagues (see Nelson, 1986) used Schank and Abelson's notion of script to study children's cognitive competence as illustrated by the children's ability to create event descriptions, to solve problems, to remember, and to reason in the context of everyday events. These researchers suggest that event representations are the basic building blocks of children's thinking (Nelson & Gruendel, 1981). Their research shows how young children are able to form scripts from repeated exposures to the same or similar events. The first time an event is experienced, the child forms a mental representation of that event. When the child experiences another similar event the two representations become fused to form a generalized event representation (Nelson & Gruendel, 1981). In Nelson's view (Nelson, 1983, 1986) basic concepts emerge from such generalized representations. Elements that occur in predictable places in events eventually are classified together as people, actions, or objects and represented as concepts separable from the original event.

Nelson (1986) indicated that events themselves have structure: they proceed according to a temporal–causal sequence, and they can be seen as hierarchically organized, in that smaller segments of activities are embedded in the whole event. A script or generalized event representation is structured in much the same way as the event and represents the event structure. However, there is no guarantee that the event representation will include everything from the event structure; thus children's representations may be lacking in certain respects. An individual's verbal description of an event is based on, though not isomorphic with, his or her representation of the event and may incompletely reflect the actual event structure.

Scripts can include subscripts in their hierarchical structure (Abelson, 1981). A restaurant script is likely to be made up of the subscripts of ordering a meal, eating, and paying. Alternate subscripts or tracks may be taken to achieve the same goal. For example, fast food restaurants have a different track for achieving the goal of buying and eating food than the track for sit-down restaurants. Abelson (1981) also distinguished strong from weak versions of scripts. Scripts and subscripts may have a temporally invariant order (strong version), such as ordering and then eating a meal in a restaurant, or they may include components that have no specified temporal order (weak version), such as eating and pitching a tent during a camping event (Nelson, 1986; see also Sonnenmeier, Chapter 10). Many events have strong and weak components. A birthday party includes some subscripts with arbitrary ordering (opening the presents can come before or after eating the cake) and some with required ordering (e.g., singing happy birthday before blowing out the candles) (Nelson, 1986).

Scripts represent culturally defined events. Adults guide children through participation in cultural events. Children can thus learn about scripts not only through observation but also as they act in adult-guided events. (See, as an example, the "greeting" script described in Crago & Eriks-Brophy, Chapter 4.)

THE LANGUAGE REFLECTING SCRIPTAL UNDERSTANDINGS

Children's knowledge and memory are typically communicated through language. Moreover, a child's language provides a window on the child's scriptal understanding.

Researchers have examined the language children use to describe events (Duchan, 1986; French, 1986; French & Nelson, 1981). Duchan (1986) identified particular linguistic elements that are tied to children's event understandings. They include semantic relations, words indicating aspect (e.g., continuing action, completed action, repetitive activity), tense markers, adverbs and adverbial phrases, and perfect tense and modal verbs.

French (1986) studied children's use of definite and indefinite articles in their event descriptions. She found that children distinguished the contexts for use of the definite article "the" from those contexts requiring the indefinite "a." They used "the" to introduce items inferable from the script, even though the items had not been previously introduced (e.g., "the teacher" when describing school events, "the cake" when describing birthday parties) and "a" when introducing noninferable specific items (e.g., "a chair," when describing a particular party). This evidence has been used to infer that children know which items are intrinsically related to events (e.g., the cake for birthday party events) and that they distinguish those from items that are less related to the event's essence (e.g., chairs for birthday party events).

Children by age three are able to describe routine events using the general pronominal forms "you" and "we" and tenseless verb forms (e.g., "you eat and drink" to describe "what you do at a restaurant") (French, 1986). Older children use the conjunctions "or," "if," and "sometimes" to indicate optional pathways in an event (French, 1986). Such terms suggest children's understanding of hypothetical situations and children's ability to describe alternative or conditional ideas. Children also often maintain the temporal order of the event structures they describe (French, 1986). If children recall some element that occurred before something already mentioned, they frequently engage in "temporal repairs," using terms such as "but first" and "before" to introduce the new element (French, 1986). Finally, children use language to achieve coherence in spatial, temporal, and participant orientations, as indicated by their use of deictic terms such as "come, go, here, there, you, I" to express a particular point of view (Duchan, 1991).

French and Nelson (1981) and French (1986) found that the language used in event descriptions is often more complex than language used at other times, suggesting that scripts support more advanced language production. Event representations also support young children's (three-year-olds) ability to describe complex logical relations such as coordination and disjunction and to engage in discourse about nonpresent events, a skill that they cannot accomplish unless talking about known events (French, 1986).

In summary, children's language reflects scripted knowledge, and scripts facilitate children's language use.

THE USE OF SCRIPTS AND FACTORS AFFECTING THEIR USE

Children's language competence is not the only mental proficiency affected by scriptal knowledge. When a task is undergirded with scriptal knowledge, children have been found to perform better in a variety of domains. Their pretend play is more coherent and better structured when they are enacting familiar events (Seidman, Nelson, & Gruendel, 1986); their dialogues are more sustained when carried out in scripted play (Nelson & Gruendel, 1979); and their recall is more lengthy, elaborate, and detailed when they are describing a familiar event (Farrar & Goodman, 1990; French 1986; Nelson & Gruendel, 1981).

Scriptal representations, like other sorts of mental representations, will function differently depending upon the contexts in which they are used. Certain circumstances facilitate scriptal use more than others. For example, children can remember and use scripts better in contexts of event enactment than they can in contexts of event recall (Price & Goodman, 1990), and they can describe events better when provided with cues from a sample episode (e.g., props or a salient participant) than without such cues (Farrar & Goodman, 1990, 1992; Smith, Ratner, & Hobart, 1987). Thus, scriptal knowledge is not static, but rather is an emergent property of an individual in interaction with her or his environmental context.

A MODEL FOR LEARNING AND USING SCRIPTS AS EVENT REPRESENTATIONS

The considerable research on scriptal learning and use among children and adults provides a basis for the formation of a theoretical model of script processing. The model could include basic principles for how typical children learn and use scripts and could offer a way of thinking about scriptal learning differences in atypical children.

Goodman (1981) has developed such a model based on her own research and that of others studying schema memory in children and adults (e.g., Nelson, 1986). In a 1980 study, Goodman showed familiar scenes to adults and children ages seven and nine. The scenes were of action events such as a picture of a woman reading a book with a potted plant next to her. She asked her subjects to remember the scene and to tell her the information in it. In free recall, her subjects reported schema-relevant information (the book) more often than schema-irrelevant information (the potted plant.) However, when shown an object from the scene along with another item similar to it (a different potted plant, a different book), children and adults recognized the picture of the original irrelevant item (the plant) better than the relevant one (the book).

Schema theory led Goodman to theorize from these findings that both adults and children use their well-formed event representations to guide their recall of the event. In so doing they structured their schemas so that information central and relevant to the schema was most accessible. In contrast, subjects store schema-irrelevant information in a separate representation that is more loosely attached to the main representation. This separate representation was hypothesized to be relatively rich in perceptual detail, probably because it takes more attentional effort to store it in the first place.

There were no age differences demonstrated in Goodman's initial studies. However, it seemed that there should be. Younger children have been shown to be more schema-dependent than adults. For example, some researchers found that younger children are more likely than older children to recall information that matches their schemas than information that does not, and that younger children were more likely than older children to intrude their expectations from the conceptual schemas into their event recall (Nelson, 1983).

What might account for the differences in attention and memory for schema-consistent and schema-inconsistent information? It seems that it is not just a function of age or even development. There was evidence for variability in memory even for children within the same age group, as well as for same-aged children across tasks. To account for such variability, Goodman (1981) developed a model of children's schema processing involving two stages. In the first stage children were hypothesized to classify events as particular instances of a known schema, concentrating on confirming what is already known. In the second it was hypothesized that children came to recognize the specificities of that particular event, concentrating on discrepancies from the typical event.

We introduce a third stage here, in which the child is in the process of developing a schema representation. The three proposed stages involved in learning and processing schemas follow.

If a schema is being formed or is not yet functioning as a coherent mental unit, it will be more difficult to process a particular experience that could fit that schema. This early stage of developing schemas is called **schema formation.**

Once formed, schemas can be used to process particular experiences. The first step in schema processing is **schema confirmation** in which a particular experience is classified as fitting a particular known schema.

After schemas have been classified through the process of schema confirmation, schema-inconsistent information is likely to be selectively attended, leading to the establishment of a somewhat separate representation in memory. This separate representation reflects **schema deployment.**

It was hypothesized by Goodman and her colleagues that when children process a particular event, the speed by which they go through the schema confirmation to deployment phases, will vary depending upon age and how well the schema is formed. Younger, less developmentally mature children should take longer to confirm their schemas. Also, the more complex the information, the harder to form a schema, and the longer it will take even mature children and adults to go from the confirmation to deployment.

Research results already in the literature offer evidence for the proposed model. Katherine Nelson and her students (Fivush, 1984; Hudson & Nelson, 1986; Nelson, 1986) found that memory for a specific autobiographical event did not develop until sufficient event memory was present. This fits the schema confirmation-deployment hypothesis in that specific events typically deviate to some extent from the prototype and thus specific autobiographical memory for such events should be formed only when the schema deployment rather than confirmation phase has been reached.

A more specific test of the hypothesis was provided in a study conducted by Farrar and Goodman in a study of script acquisition (Farrar & Goodman, 1992). The method involved exposing children to unfamiliar events. Specifically, the authors set up an event consisting of a series of "standard activities" for the children to participate in and varied the number of times the children experienced this entire event (one vs. three times). They then introduced to children a "deviation event" consisting of activities with inconsistent or discrepant information relative to the standard event. The new activities were called "deviation activities." No child experienced more than one deviation event.

The activities carried out for standard events consisted of the child and an adult guide using two toy animals to perform a set of four activities. For example, one activity involved the child and adult having a frog and rabbit puppet jumping over a fence; another involved the child and adult playing pop-up with a toy bear and squirrel. There were three types of deviations: (1) changes in the animals and actions (e.g., having a toy dog and pig swinging on the pop-up set) (2) changes in the activity (e.g., building toys out of Legos instead of using the pop-up set) and (3) changes in the sequence

TABLE 9-1 Manipulations of visits and exposure to event conditions for the four groups

Groups	ORDER OF VISIT TYPES FOR EACH GROUP			
	Day 1	Day 2	Day 3	Day 4
One-visit standard group	Standard event	—	—	—
One-visit deviation group	Deviation event	—	—	—
Two-visit group	Standard event	Deviation event		
Four-visit group	Standard event	Standard event	Standard event	Deviation event

Adapted from M. J. Farrar and G. S. Goodman (1992). Developmental changes in event memory. *Child Development, 63,* 173–187, with permission of the Society for Research in Child Development.

of two of the events (e.g., changing the order so that the fence-jumping activity came after the pop-up activity).

The subjects were 32 four-year-old and 32 seven-year-old typically developing children. There were eight children from each age group participating in each of four treatment groups.

The treatment groups are indicated in Table 9-1. The one-visit standard group experienced the four different standard events, one time each. Similarly, the one-visit deviation group experienced four deviation events, one time each. These groups provided the baseline information about memory for each event. They also provided information about children's memory for events experienced only one time, rather than repeatedly.

The two-visit group experienced both the four standard and four deviation events, one time each. With such limited exposure to the standard event, the children should have been in the process of forming a schema for that event. The four-visit group had three experiences with each of the same standard event before exposure to the deviation event.

A week after experiencing the last event, all children were interviewed by a person they had never met. They were asked general questions about what happened on particular visits, allowing for their free recall of the four activities within an event. There were two contexts in which the questions were asked, one in a room separate from that in which the activities were experienced (free recall) and one in the same room where they experienced the activities (contextual recall). Children's responses were scored for whether they remembered each activity as a whole (activity recall, "we played pop-up") and whether they remembered the details (props, animals, actions) of the activities (activity instantiations).

As shown in Table 9-2, seven-year-olds recalled more activities and details than the four-year-olds. Children from both age groups who experienced one standard visit recalled the activities and details about as well as

TABLE 9-2 Mean proportion of correct event information recalled about the standard visit (collapsed over free and contextual recall tests) as a function of age group and event condition

	STANDARD ONE VISIT	TWO VISITS (ONE STANDARD, ONE DEVIATION VISIT)	FOUR VISITS (ONE DEVIATION VISIT)
Activity Recall			
4-year-olds	.55	.41	.53
7-year-olds	.80	.71	.88
Activity Instantiations			
4-year-olds	.36	.24	.31
7-year-olds	.62	.47	.63

children who experienced three standard visits. These results indicate how easily and quickly children establish at least rudimentary event representations.

The consistent dip in performance between one-visit and two-visit groups for both age levels indicates that children who had two visits did not remember the standard visit as well as those with one visit. This may have been due to the creation of confusion between standard and deviation event types for children in the two-visit group who experienced both standard and deviation events. Children in the four-visit group did as well as those in the one-visit group, indicating that additional standard visits helped cancel the negative effects of the deviation event. The U-shaped function was characteristic of children's performance on both recall conditions (free and contextual).

As shown in Table 9-3, the more experience children had with the standard visit, the poorer their recall of the deviation visit. The decline in recall of the deviation events is true for both age groups and for recall of activities as well as details. This consistent result can be interpreted as a reflection of the emergence of the standard event as the primary memory representation, showing that children as young as four are able to form generalized event representations for events experienced only three times.

The tasks were designed to allow for a determination of the degree of feature substitution in children's recall (features being activities, props, or animals). For example, children who had experienced the standard event and the deviation event needed to include standard event features to correctly recall the elements of the standard event. Table 9-4 indicates that standard features were mentioned correctly in the recall of standard events, and incorrectly in the recall of deviation events. This "inclusion error effect" for the deviation event was similar for both age groups (28 percent for four-year-olds, 32 percent for seven-year-olds). However, four-year-olds included as

TABLE 9-3 Mean proportion of correct event information recalled about the deviation visit (collapsed over free and contextual recall tests) as a function of age group and event condition

	ONE DEVIATION VISIT	TWO VISITS (ONE STANDARD, ONE DEVIATION VISIT)	FOUR VISITS (ONE DEVIATION VISIT)
Activity Recall			
4-year-olds	.56	.49	.37
7-year-olds	.79	.82	.69
Activity Instantiations			
4-year-olds	.34	.29	.20
7-year-olds	.60	.52	.45

many standard features in their recall of the standard events as they did in their recall of the deviation event, whereas the seven-year olds seemed to be making a distinction between the two events.

Measures were also made of the degree to which features of the deviation visit intruded, incorrectly, in children's recall of the standard visit. As seen in Table 9-5, this intrusion was minimal for both groups of children, 17 percent of four-year-old responses, and 11 percent of the responses of the seven-year-olds. Table 9-5 also compares children's incorrect recall of deviation event features when remembering standard events, with children's correct recollection of deviation event features for deviation events. Four-year-olds included deviation event features equally in their recall of standard as well as deviation events, whereas seven-year-olds were able to better remember the idiosyncrasies of the deviation event, suggesting that they stored them separately in memory, apart from their general event representation of standard events.

Thus, older children were better able than younger children to separate the visits in memory. Four-year-olds did not seem to make as much of a

TABLE 9-4 Mean proportion of standard event features included by children in recall of the standard event and the deviation event as a function of age group (collapsed across free and contextual recall tests)

	EVENT TYPE	
Age Group	Standard Event [a]	Deviation Event [b]
4-year-olds	.25	.28
7-year-olds	.50	.32

[a] Correct recall of standard event features as having occurred during the standard event
[b] Incorrect recall of standard event features as having occurred during the deviation event

TABLE 9-5 Mean proportion of deviation event features included by children in recall of the standard event and the deviation event as a function of age group (collapsed across free and contextual recall tests)

	EVENT TYPE	
Age Group	Standard Event [a]	Deviation Event [b]
4-year-olds	.17	.19
7-year-olds	.11	.35

[a]Incorrect recall of deviation event features as having occurred during the standard event
[b]Correct recall of deviation event features as having occurred during the deviation event

distinction between the two types of events, as evidenced by their inclusion of features of deviant events in their standard event descriptions, as well as their standard event features in their descriptions of deviant events.

Finally, Farrar and Goodman analyzed their data to determine whether the children's abilities to separate standard events from deviation events differed depending upon the child's amount of experience with the events. The confirmation–deployment hypothesis would predict that recall of both standard and deviation event details would improve as children develop a generalized representation of the standard event, and as they develop a separate memory for particular experiences that do not fit that generalized representation.

As shown in Table 9-6, the number of details recalled from the standard and deviant activities was virtually equivalent for children from both age groups exposed to each event once. This suggests that with only two visits children did not have enough experience to treat the events of the standard visit as general, and different from the deviation events. Seven-year-olds in the two-visit group included the same number of deviation features in their recall of the deviation visit as they did the standard visit. However, those seven-year-olds with additional experience with the standard activities, the four-visit group, were able to remember the deviation details for deviation events and did not include them in their recall of standard events. The four-

TABLE 9-6 Mean proportion recall of new activity instantiations (deviation details) as a function of age group, event type, and amount of event experience (collapsed across free and contextual recall tests)

	TWO-VISIT GROUP		FOUR-VISIT GROUP	
	Standard Event	Deviation Event	Standard Event	Deviation Event
4-year-olds	.03	.09	.25	.09
7-year-olds	.20	.20	.06	.32

year-olds, on the other hand, incorrectly included more details of deviation events in their description of standard events than they did in the deviation events, evidencing considerable confusion.

Taken together, these findings indicate that younger children organize their memory for general and specific event episodes, but their organization is at times different from that of older children, at least while learning about an event. Four-year-olds in the Farrar and Goodman (1992) study had a single, more or less combined representation for both standard and deviation events, as evidenced by their confusion about the details of particular events. Seven-year-olds, in contrast, did a better job of establishing distinct memories for the two types of events, perhaps because they were able to more effectively establish an event representation with which to mentally contrast the deviation visit.

WHAT MAY BE OCURRING WITH CHILDREN WHO HAVE TROUBLE FORMING SCRIPTS

Current assessment and intervention approaches for use with children who have language learning problems often do not include the children's event representations as an area of focus. Instead, existing approaches treat children's language as separate from event knowledge. Children who do not talk during routine activities may be having difficulty understanding what is going on. In these cases, their difficulty may not be one of vocabulary or syntax but rather one of not understanding the event (see Shultz, 1979, for an example of a child who is regarded by her teacher as incompetent because she did not understand how to play tic-tac-toe).

The distinction among formation, confirmation, and deployment can be used as a way to organize assessment and intervention procedures. We might ask, for example, if a child has experienced an event previously, and if so, how often. More experience with an event can give a child a better grounding for using language during the event and for describing the event to someone else. Or we might ask whether the child has an event representation that matches the conventional representations. Perhaps certain aspects of events, such as where people are sitting, or how objects are arranged, are relevant to the individual child's construction of an event, and irrelevant in a conventional representation (Duchan, 1991). This would lead the child to classify new instances of the event differently, resulting in a difference in schema confirmation. Or we might ask whether the child is flexible in his or her acceptance of deviant aspects of an event. This lack of acceptance, sometimes called rigidity or preservation of sameness (see Duchan, Chapter 11) could lead to a problem in schema deployment in which new details are emotionally rejected, thus blocking children's ability to represent novel aspects of familiar events. Finally, we could ask if some children are so preoccupied with emotional issues activated by the event itself, the social interaction of discussing it later, or general events in their homelife that their concentration on event processing or event retrieval is disrupted.

An example of how the model presented here might be used is offered in the next chapter in which Sonnenmeier presents an intervention approach that is sensitive to different stages of children's scriptal processing. Future research will provide a test of the model's usefulness for depicting what children with learning problems know about their world, and how event knowledge affects all children's everyday understanding, social competence, learning, memory, and language development.

REFERENCES

Abelson, R. P. (1981). Psychological status of the script concept. *American Psychologist, 36* (7), 715–729.

Bartlett, F. C. (1932). *Remembering: A study in experimental and social psychology.* New York: Cambridge University Press.

Bruner, J. (1983). The acquisition of pragmatic commitments. In R. Golinkoff (Ed.), *The transition from prelinguistic to linguistic communication.* Hillsdale, NJ: Lawrence Erlbaum.

Duchan, J. (1986). Learning to describe events. *Topics in Language Disorders, 6,* 27–36.

Duchan, J. (1991). Everyday events: Their role in language assessment and intervention. In T. Gallagher (Ed.), *Pragmatics of language: Clinical practice issues.* San Diego, CA: Singular Publishing Company.

Farrar, J., & Goodman, G. (1990). Developmental differences in the relation between scripts and episodic memory: Do they exist? In R. Fivush & J. Hudson (Eds.), *Knowing and remembering in young children* (pp. 30–64). New York: Cambridge University Press.

Farrar, J., & Goodman, G. (1992). Developmental changes in event memory. *Child Development, 63,* 173–187.

Fivush, R. (1984). Learning about school: The development of kindergartners' school scripts. *Child Development, 55,* 1679–1709.

French, L. A. (1986). The language of events. In K. Nelson (Ed.), *Event knowledge: Structure and function in development.* Hillsdale, NJ: Lawrence Erlbaum.

French, L. A., & Nelson, K. (1981). Temporal knowledge expressed in preschoolers' descriptions of familiar activites. *Papers and Reports on Child Language Development, 20,* 61–69.

Goodman, G. (1980). Picture memory: How the action schema affects retention. *Cognitive Psychology, 12,* 473–495.

Goodman, G. (1981). *Schema-confirmation and schema-deployment.* Unpublished manuscript.

Hudson, J., & Nelson, K. (1986). Repeated encounters of a similar kind: Effects of familiarity on children's autobiographical memory. *Child Development, 57,* 253–271.

Lund, N., & Duchan, J. (1993). *Assessing children's language in naturalistic contexts,* 3rd ed. Englewood Cliffs, NJ: Prentice Hall.

Mandler, J. (1984). *Stories, scripts, and scenes: Aspects of schema theory.* Hillsdale, NJ: Lawrence Erlbaum.

Mandler, J. M. (1979). Categorical and schematic organization in memory. In C. R. Puff (Ed.), *Memory organization and structure* (pp. 259–299). New York: Academic Press.

Nelson, K. (1983). The derivation of concepts and categories from event representations. In E. Scholnick (Ed.), *New trends in conceptual representation: Challenges to Piaget's theory?* Hillsdale, NJ: Lawrence Erlbaum.

Nelson, K. (Ed.). (1986). *Event knowledge: Structure and function in development.* Hillsdale, NJ: Lawrence Erlbaum.

Nelson, K., & Gruendel, J. (1979). At morning it's lunchtime: A scriptal view of children's dialogues. *Discourse Processes, 2,* 73–94.

Nelson, K., & Gruendel, J. (1981). Generalized event representations: Basic building blocks of cognitive development. In M. E. Lamb & A. L. Brown (Eds.), *Advances in developmental psychology* (Vol. 1, pp. 131–158). Hillsdale, NJ: Lawrence Erlbaum.

Price, D., & Goodman, G. (1990). Visiting the wizard: Children's memory for a recurring event. *Child Development, 61,* 664–680.

Rumelhart, D. (1980). Schemata: The building blocks of cognition. In R. Spiro, B. Bruce, & W. Brewer (Eds.), *Theoretical issues in reading comprehension.* Hillsdale, NJ: Lawrence Erlbaum.

Schank, R., & Abelson, R. (1977). *Scripts, plans, goals, and understanding.* Hillsdale, NJ: Lawrence Erlbaum.

Shultz, J. (1979). It's not whether you win or lose, it's how you play the game. In O. Garnica & M. King (Eds.), *Language, children, and society.* Elmsford, NY: Pergamon Press.

Seidman, S., Nelson, K., & Gruendel, J. (1986). Make believe scripts: The transformation of ERs in fantasy. In K. Nelson (Ed.), *Event knowledge: Structure and function in development.* Hillsdale, NJ: Lawrence Erlbaum.

Smith, B., Ratner, H. H., & Hobart, C. (1987). The role of cueing and organization in children's memory for events. *Journal of Experimental Child Psychology, 44,* 1–24.

Tulving, E. (1972). Episodic and semantic memory. In E. Tulving & W. Donaldson (Eds.), *Organization of memory* (pp. 381–403). New York: Academic Press.

chapter 10

SCRIPT-BASED LANGUAGE INTERVENTION:
Learning to Participate in Life Events

Rae M. Sonnenmeier

INTRODUCTION

The ultimate and inherently pragmatic goal of any language intervention program is for children to use language in the context of everyday life events. Goodman, Duchan, and Sonnenmeier (Chapter 9) point out that research in the area of cognitive psychology has highlighted the role scriptal knowledge plays in children's understanding of such everyday events (see also, Nelson, 1986). Scripts support children's ability to participate, describe, and recall familiar events as well as to use language during such events.

It is through participation in everyday experiences that children learn a particular view of the world and develop the knowledge base from which they may make sense out of new experiences. If children are confronted with a novel event, it seems reasonable that they will attempt to make sense out of it and participate in it based on prior experiences. As Goodman, et al. (Chapter 9) suggests, children are likely to "confirm" the familiar aspects of currently experienced or remembered events and then to "deploy" a variation of the typical event structure for understanding or remembering novel aspects. The general sequence for what you do at Friendly's is not all that different from what you do at Pizza Hut: You go to the restaurant, you wait for someone to seat you, you look at the menu, you tell the waiter or waitress what you want to eat, and so forth. What is different is what you might order or the way in which you eat, given the difference in the food items. Once a child recognizes or confirms the similarity in the two events, then knowing what to do or say in either is not difficult. On the other hand, children who have not abstracted the generalized event representation for "restaurant," or who have a specific event representation for restaurant based on Pizza Hut only, may not be able to rely on previous experiences in order to successfully participate in a new event, such as going to Friendly's. Children often get upset when the event does not proceed as expected. In these cases, teachers, clinicians, or parents help children make comparisons across similar events and understand different versions of the same event. Through repeated experiences children will be better able to abstract a more generalized event representation, which leads to greater understanding and better performance in event-based life experiences.

Children's successful participation in events with others also depends on how similar their event representations are to those of their interactants. Differences in two interactants' understanding of a particular event can lead to differences in how they participate in the event and then to "miscommunications." Often we are surprised when children do not do something in the way we would. Imagine a child who has a narrow representation of an event or does not have prior experience with the event. Such children appear incompetent or incorrigible on occasions when knowledge of that event is required.

This chapter is an attempt to blend clinical practice with the theoretical perspective of scripts in order to help children learn and use event knowledge. The design of the intervention approach has evolved, with theory guiding practice and practice creating questions for the theoretical literature to help answer. A framework will be presented for planning and implementing script-based intervention with preschool children who exhibit various handicapping conditions (language delay, autism, Down syndrome, developmental delays, etc.). The intervention approach focuses on the expansion of children's event knowledge to support their expressive language abilities during familiar daily routines, such as feeding a baby, as well as during less familiar community-based events, such as going to a restaurant.

THE USE OF EVERYDAY EVENTS IN CLINICAL PRACTICE

When practitioners learned of the role of pragmatics in language acquisition, they began designing language interventions that took place in naturally occurring contexts. Particularly influential was Bruner's work, which revealed the importance of routines in language learning for typical children (Bruner, 1975; Ninio & Bruner, 1978; Ratner & Bruner, 1978). Bruner and his colleagues showed that children learn language through active participation in familiar events, not by passive observation alone. Taking these results and applying them to language teaching, practitioners discarded worksheets and drill activities in favor of more naturalistic contexts such as play (Culatta, 1984; DeMaio, 1984; Weitzner-Lin, Sonnenmeier, & Murphy, 1983) and book-reading (Kirchner, 1991). Routines and sociodramatic play activities were used as vehicles for encouraging children's use of language in familiar contexts (Duchan & Weitzner-Lin, 1987; Snyder-McLean, Solomonson, McLean, & Sack, 1984).

The idea of encouraging language in "natural" contexts has gained increased importance as clinicians have moved into classrooms, since these are the naturally occurring everyday contexts requiring children's participation. Integrated school settings provide endless opportunities for encouraging language use by children with special needs as they relate to their typical peers. The focus has changed from carrying out intervention in a clinician–child dyad to helping children communicate with their peers in the activities in which they participate throughout the day. Clinicians and teachers focus on strategies for encouraging typical peers to act as models for what to say and do in the activities.

It is in the context of integrated programs that it becomes obvious that many children with special needs have different views of the world than those of their typical peers. There are children who scream or tantrum when the class transitions to new activities or goes to new places in the community. Clinicians and teachers struggle to figure out how to help children make sense of their world so that they can successfully participate in play and other activities with their peers, as well as become effective communicators.

One means for providing children with practice on what to do in daily events is through directed pretend play or "scripted play" (Fey, 1986, p. 214). Once children become familiar with an event through play, they can expand their use of language in real-life contexts.

Through observation and documented progress, programs built around scripted events have been found to be successful in encouraging children's use of language (Constable, 1986). Success is often attributed to the repetition provided and the increased familiarity with the activities. Teaching children what to say during pretend play is one step to effective communication but what else might children be learning as they participate in pretend play? The literature on scripts and events, including the work of Nelson (1986), Westby (1988), Constable (1983, 1986) and Snyder-McLean, et al. (1984) provide a rich account of aspects of events that children learn from scripted play activities.

WHAT CHILDREN LEARN BY PARTICIPATING
IN EVERYDAY EVENTS

Bruner and his colleagues (Bruner, 1975; Bruner & Sherwood, 1976; Ninio & Bruner, 1978; Ratner & Bruner, 1978) found that the early routines carried out between infants and their caregivers provide opportunities for learning features that occur across many routine events. These features include understanding that a routine event has a predictable sequence, that language is used at particular points within that event, that there are specific roles that interactants may play within the event, and that these roles are reciprocal (Ratner & Bruner, 1978). Such routines set the stage for learning about events in general and provide a supportive context in which children may slowly expand upon the range of language forms and functions they are able to express.

As children grow older, they add to their knowledge of routines to develop an understanding of longer, more complex, and varying events. For example, children initially learn to assume responsibility in a social game such as peek-a-boo. They learn about turn taking and the interdependence of participants. As children observe and participate in everyday events, such as bathing or mealtime, they build on their knowledge of role relationships acquired during routines. As their experiences begin to include events in the community, this knowledge further develops to include more specified roles such as customer and waitress, ticket seller, and so on. Such knowledge has been described as a part of what Nelson and Gruendel (1981) called "generalized event representations," namely, "scripts" (see Goodman et al., Chapter 9, for a review).

Schank and Abelson (1977) originally described scripts as being "made up of slots and requirements about what can fill those slots" (p. 41). Nelson and Gruendel (1981) used the slot notion of Schank and Abelson (1977) in their study of children's knowledge acquisition. They characterized scripts as "general schemas or frames within which variable elements may be inserted in appropriate contexts" (p. 131). Knowledge of what can fill a slot, according to Nelson (1986), includes expanding on the notions of the various roles individuals can assume within an event, the objects that are typically used, the possible sequence of actions that may be based on the temporal and causal relationships, as well as goals within the event and the plans for accomplishing these goals.

Scriptal knowledge forms the conceptual representation for personal experiences, which organizes individuals' knowledge base about events as well as their thoughts and language relevant to these events. This knowledge allows individuals to form expectations for what will happen in an event, supporting their ability to participate within it. Furthermore, and what is important to language interventionists, scripts provide support for the use of language during events, as well as when describing what typically happens in a particular event.

Nelson and Gruendel (1979) found that scripts also provide a structure for children's conversations during play and that children use their scriptal knowledge to sustain these conversations. Thus, shared scriptal knowledge allows children to carry on a pretend telephone conversation regarding the negotiation of plans for dinner, a conversation based on their knowledge of how such events typically go. Their knowledge of what to say in the conversation is also a reflection of their understanding of the various roles within the script.

Since scripts describe culturally defined events that have been given conventional labels (Nelson, 1986), the original notions of scripts seemed to suggest that event representations are similar for members of the same culture—that there might be something such as a "culturally agreed upon script" for particular events. Adults guide children's participation in cultural events. In this way children learn conventional ways of thinking about and participating in their culture's activities.

It has been found that individuals may develop a different sense of an event depending on their role within the event (Duchan, 1991). Ross and Berg (1990) reported on the individual differences reflected in adults' descriptions of events based on their particular role. For example, an airplane pilot has a very different script for an airport event than does a passenger. The types of experiences one has had in an event also account for individual differences. Thus, someone who travels a great deal may include "luggage getting lost" as part of his or her script whereas someone else may not. This points out the variability that exists between individuals and the importance of experience in the formation of a script. This is a crucial notion in understanding children's scriptal knowledge, particularly children who may pay attention to different aspects of events. As a result, they probably form an idiosyncratic event representation which then leads them to participate in events differently than others might, based on having different expectations about the event.

Children's underlying knowledge of scripts has primarily been studied by examining their descriptions of events (Nelson & Gruendel, 1981). Researchers assume that particular scriptal elements have been conceptually established if they occur as part of a child's event description. However, some researchers have found that children are better able to recall elements of a script when given contextual support such as that provided by event enactments (Farrar & Goodman, 1990, 1992; Smith, Ratner, & Hobart, 1987). Understanding that children are able to demonstrate what they know about events through enactments has lead to assessment and intervention procedures that emphasize the incorporation of event knowledge.

In summary, it has been found that children's acquisition of event knowledge consists of their learning a variety of features. For example, children learn about role relationships, action sequences, and object use that are included in their event representations. The features serve not only as structure for particular events but also as abstract "slots" that allow children to understand event structure in general. Children use their knowledge of event structure to support their participation and use of language during events. In addition, children come to understand, through adult guidance, cultural conventions regarding events.

SUPPORT FOR THE USE OF A SCRIPT-BASED APPROACH TO LANGUAGE ASSESSMENT AND INTERVENTION

The use of a script-based approach to language assessment and intervention has been promoted by various researchers (Constable, 1983, 1986; Culatta, Chapter 8; Duchan, 1991; Duchan & Weitzner-Lin, 1987; Snyder-McLean et al., 1984; Westby, 1980, 1988). Westby (1980, 1988) provides a scale for assessing children's play skills that can be used to gain insight into their conceptual understanding of the physical world as well as their understanding of social interactions within familiar events. Westby (1980) used her Symbolic Play Scale with children exhibiting various handicapping conditions, including autism, mental retardation, attention-deficit disorders, and speech/language impairments. She found children with disabilities played differently from their typical peers and noted that the variability was related to the elements of scripts used in the children's play. In the revision of her play scale, Westby (1988) includes assessment of scriptal elements as follows:

1. The relationships between self and others and the ability to adopt the ROLES of others in pretend activities
2. The organization of play themes, emphasizing the SEQUENCE of actions and overall coherence of play events
3. The content of the scripts, emphasizing the overall GOAL or theme of the play event
4. The ideas about how OBJECTS are used within the events, including the trend for play to occur with decreasing environmental support or changing reliance on props (from realistic, to abstract, to invented)

Examiners can use Westby's scale to assess children's development of all four dimensions (Westby, 1988). This provides a format for determining what aspects of the event a child knows and uses in interactions as well as identifying potential areas in which the child's event knowledge may be different from that of others. The findings based on use of this scale have specific intervention implications. For example, those children who depend on others for the organization of their play could benefit from specific interventions designed to increase their understanding of the events upon which the play is based.

Snyder-McLean et al. (1984) suggest that children with delayed language may not always attend to the most relevant features of an event, at least those most relevant for an adult. Constable (1983) recommends providing perceptual support to highlight relevant aspects of events that foster language learning. Such perceptual support includes making available relevant objects.

Constable (1983, 1986) and Snyder-McLean et al. (1984) suggest that scripts provide a social context for learning as well as a way for children to learn about actors, objects, and actions within the event. They see the building of scripts with children as creating a shared knowledge base between the child and the interactant, increasing the child's attention to relevant or script-consistent information, thereby enhancing overall communicative competence.

Snyder-McLean and colleagues (1984) have devised scripted intervention through the use of what they call "joint action routines." They define a joint action routine as

> a ritualized interaction pattern, involving joint action, unified by a specific theme or goal, which follows a logical sequence, including a clear beginning point, and in which each participant plays a recognizable role, with specific response expectancies, that is essential to the successful completion of that sequence. (p. 214)

These authors regard joint action routines as being somewhere between Bruner's tightly formatted routines and social games and Nelson's more loosely structured scripts. Similar to the tightly formatted routines, joint action routines provide a "scaffold" (Bruner, 1975) that supports the child's use of language in an event. Additionally, such routines may provide an opportunity to assist a child who may have a different view of the world in gaining an understanding of the culturally accepted views of events (Snyder-McLean et al., 1984). Furthermore, such communicative contexts are easily incorporated into classroom contexts and allow for the opportunity to encourage meaningful interactions between children with language impairments and their peers. Snyder-McLean et al. (1984) argue that the features present in these early routines can be useful in planning intervention programs for young as well as older children at a prelinguistic or a beginning stage in their language learning.

Duchan and Weitzner-Lin (1987) advocate for the use of specific events to facilitate children's use of particular language forms and functions. They present a framework for planning events such as storytelling to develop discourse skills, routines for encouraging participation and turn taking, and sociodramatic play for enhancing conversational competence.

Most of the approaches highlight the need for children to possess event knowledge, which then supports their use of language in specific contexts. Constable (1983, 1986) emphasizes the use of context to increase children's understanding and use of specific linguistic forms. Snyder-McLean et al. (1984) and Duchan and Weitzner-Lin (1987) promote the use of particular events for the learning of specific pragmatic and discourse skills. However, events need to be emphasized in intervention not simply as vehicles for facilitating language use and language form, but for emphasizing event knowledge in and of itself. The approach of script-based intervention developed here treats event knowledge in its own right and not just as a means for learning language.

A FRAMEWORK FOR PLANNING SCRIPT-BASED PLAY EVENTS

So how might we teach children generalized event representations? By designing play and real-life situations that include elements of scripts, clinicians can help children develop the knowledge they need to support their participation in events. While the use of sociodramatic play is not new to language interventionists, using play to teach children event knowledge is. When targeting event representations as a goal, interventionists need to do more than set out materials and model appropriate language forms in context. They also need to consider:

1. Overall organization of the event
2. Roles of participants and the perspective of the event from given roles
3. Temporal relationships (sequence)
4. Causal relationships (goals and plans)
5. Objects related to the event

The adult begins by providing at least one version of how to participate in the event, highlighting specific aspects of the event. The formation–confirmation–deployment hypothesis developed by Goodman et al. (Chapter 9) has application here. The event presented will be familiar to some children, allowing them to confirm the aspects of the events that they know and can recall. Particular events may never have been experienced by some children or may have been experienced in very different ways. These children will engage in the process of forming an event representation. Other children may recognize the events and are able to note variations of the events, utilizing their deployment skills. Thus, a particular enactment of an event may focus on different skills for different children. For the children who seem to have a different view of the event, the same demonstration offers them experience in a series of repeated experiences that could help them develop an event representation.

Clinicians and teachers using a scriptal approach to intervention need to consider elements of events when planning structured play events. Certain events emphasize particular aspects of scriptal knowledge; some provide a focus on the sequence, while others require attention to roles and various perspectives based on roles.

Initially, it is beneficial to involve the child in event sequences congruent with his or her role or perspective. For example, when going to the restaurant, the child would always be in the customer role; when going to the doctor, in the patient role. It is useful to point out to the children that the roles are often similar across many events. Children need to learn the familiar role of "customer," whether it be at a grocery store, shoe store, or restaurant, or when purchasing a ticket for a movie. At the same time, children need to learn about the role of "worker," or the person who can provide the service, whether it be a cashier, waiter, or ticket seller. Through repeated experiences children will learn to take on a different perspective within the event and assume a less familiar role.

In addition, some actions and event sequences can be incorporated into different events. For example, going somewhere in the community usually involves "getting ready," which may include getting dressed and checking to make sure we have enough money before driving to our destination. Such "subscripts" (Abelson, 1981) can be included regularly in event reenactments to support children's participation in the familiar portions of the events. "Families" can "drive" pretend cars to stores or restaurants, building in generalization across events. Over time, variations in subscripts can be introduced; sometimes the family could walk or take a bus to the store. The variations can be used to help children learn about new events.

Some events do not emphasize roles at all. For example, a camping event focuses on the things you do while camping but not so much on *who* is doing *what;* it tends to be a group effort. Such an event is really a combination of many subscripts, including shopping for food, packing, traveling to the campsite, hiking, cooking, bedtime, and so on. It is likely that children will recognize some of the subscripts embedded in the event and incorporate this information to participate in the "camping" event. In addition, the temporal and causal sequencing of some subscripts matters, such as making the fire in order to cook dinner. On the other hand, the sequence of other subscripts in a camping event is more arbitrary; it does not matter if you go for a hike before or after lunch.

Clinicians and teachers can take advantage of the similarities in roles and action sequences and build upon children's previous experiences to help them learn about new events. In this way, adults guide children in the process of confirming the subscripts as familiar and encourage the deployment effect in the recognition of variations or novel aspects of the subscripts. The focus of a selected scripted play activity might be to demonstrate any one or more of the following: possible event sequences, roles for the participants, goals and plans for fulfilling those goals, and ways of using the materials.

Early in the school year, events can be chosen that are familiar to the children, such as the daily events of bathtime, dressing, feeding, and perhaps bookreading. Table 10-1 presents a list of events grouped by theme that may be rehearsed during scripted play. Children can rely on their own experiences

TABLE 10-1   Familiar Events That May Be Rehearsed During Scripted Play

Family Routines
  bedtime
  mealtime
  bathtime
  birthday party
Restaurants
  ice cream parlor
  pizza parlor
  fast food restaurant
Stores
  bakery
  grocery store
  shoe store
  post office
Medical Needs
  doctor/hospital
  dentist
  veterinarian
Travel Events
  camping
  airport
  train station
  space ship travel

and reenact these experiences with realistic materials and dolls. Over time, these experiences can be built upon to include occasional events within the family or the community, such as going to a birthday party or going to the grocery store or a restaurant. Realistic materials and even real food items can act as cues for relevant elements of the event, what Constable (1983) calls "providing perceptual support." Field trips to the community can provide real-life experience from which children can draw. Gradually, events can be introduced with which children have even less experience, such as going to the doctor or dentist, or perhaps no experience, such as taking a trip on a bus or airplane or going camping.

The "scripted play" time itself has a specific overall structure related to daily classroom routines which children come to expect over time. At the beginning of the school year, the play event can be specifically described to the children. First, the children sit and watch as an adult introduces the materials and how they can be used in the event. Likewise, the adult can review the subscripts that later will be combined into the whole event. Then the adult can model the event sequence from the beginning to the end and narrate the actions for the event while going through it. This offers the opportunity to model language use and language forms related to the event. Once the demonstration is completed, the adult can point out differences or variations for the children to pay attention to in the enactment. Then children

FIGURE 10-1 Lesson Plan: Grocery Store

A. Event Description
1. Set up of the Room

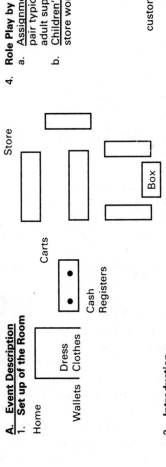

(Diagram labels: Home, Dress Clothes, Wallets, Carts, Cash Registers, Store, Box)

2. Introduction
Adult explains the focus of the "playgroup" and asks children what they know about the event

3. Adult Demonstration of "Customer Role"
a. Getting Ready to Go to the Store
  put on coat
  check to make sure you have enough money
  check the shopping list (review list with group)
  walk to the store
b. At the Store
  get a shopping cart
  look at the list and look for items on shelves
  ask store worker for help in finding items
  check-out/pay for food
  help bag items
c. Go Home

4. Role Play by Children:
a. Assignment of Roles (store worker, customer)
  pair typical child with child with special needs
  adult supports children in respective roles
b. Children's Enactment of the Scripted Event
  store worker—stock shelves
       open store
       help customers find items
       check-out/cash register
       bag items
       take money
       close store
  customer—get dressed and get money
       walk to store
       look for items on the list
       ask store workers for help with items not found
       check-out and give money to cashiers
       take items and go home.
c. Switch Roles and Reenact

5. Review Event: event descriptions
6. Free play: (next day)
set out materials for children to reenact event with minimal adult support

B. Objectives

Group Objectives (typical children):
1. to assume a pretend role (cashier, customer)
2. to follow and participate in the event sequence
3. to use vocabulary related to the event
4. to engage in conversations related to the event
5. to coherently describe the event

Individualized Objectives (delayed language):
1. to assume a pretend role (cashier) with minimal support
2. to follow and participate in the event sequence with minimal verbal cues from peers and/or adults
3. to use vocabulary related to the event
4. to initiate verbal requests to a peer for needed items

Individualized Objectives (autistic):
1. to assume a familiar role (customer) with modeling and support from a peer or an adult
2. to participate in a joint activity with a peer given modeling and verbal cues by the peer or adult
3. to follow subparts of the event sequence (e.g., getting ready) with minimal support
4. to direct language to a peer given redirection cues
5. to use 3–4 word phrases to comment given verbal or sign cues

C. Strategies

General Group Strategies
1. model vocabulary using signs for visual support
2. expansion of child utterances to add missing words (e.g., "I go home" – "I'm going home")
3. redirection to interact with peers
4. provide simple phrases for typical peers to use as models for children with special needs
5. clearly label roles and responsibilities related to roles
6. fade adult support; observe rather than interact; redirect as needed

Individualized Strategies
1. use general strategies
2. during freeplay, redirect to play with materials
3. encourage child to assume a particular role
4. fade verbal support as much as possible

Individualized Strategies
1. engage in using materials first
2. once engaged, redirect to peers' actions and utterances
3. use sign cues to encourage commenting on actions and/or event

are assigned specific roles. The child at first should be assigned to the role that he or she would typically be in, such as the customer role. The child with special needs can also be paired with a typical peer who knows the event better. The peer can model what to do and say in the event. The adult can provide varying levels of support for the children, from modeling the roles to providing verbal cues for what to do next. After the children have enacted the event, the adults can review with the children what they did, facilitating event description skills. Finally, the next morning during free play, the materials can be set out again and children can have the opportunity to reenact the event on their own terms. This offers the opportunity to assess the children's developing event representation as well as their use of language during the event.

A sample lesson plan for a "Grocery Store" scripted-play event is presented in Figure 10–1 (pp. 144–45). Section A describes the overall sequence of the play event. A diagram for how the classroom could be arranged is shown. An outline is presented for the adult demonstration of the event sequence and the role play by the children. The event sequences emphasized are based on the roles of customer or store worker, taking into account the difference in perspective based on the roles. This could be used to highlight role relationships as necessary.

Section B includes examples of objectives that could be focused on in this event. Group objectives are listed for typically developing children and are somewhat general. Two sets of individualized objectives are presented, one set for a child with delayed language development, and one set for a child with autism. Objectives emphasize the use of event knowledge, including assuming a specific role and participating in event sequences. Additional objectives focus on the use of language within the event to request needed items, comment, and interact and/or converse with peers.

Section C outlines strategies that may be used by teachers and clinicians to encourage the development of event knowledge and use of the specific skills targeted by the objectives. General strategies include modeling and labeling roles, redirection cues to focus attention on peer actions and use of language, and expansions related to utterances spoken by the children. Individualized strategies emphasize experience and adult support to encourage understanding of the event and its components.

CONCLUSION

The framework presented here for planning scripted events originated from my clinical practice. I initially designed an intervention program to teach children language in familiar everyday contexts, following the ideas already in clinical practice regarding the importance of events (Snyder-McLean et al., 1984; Ratner & Bruner, 1978). It became apparent that children could not just memorize "lines of a script." Their understanding of the specific roles and the sequence of the event also seemed important and allowed them to use language more productively. Turning back to the theoretical literature, I found an account of children's event representations that highlighted a set of components including roles and event sequences (Nelson, 1986). Further, I discovered the notion of "subscripts" (Abelson, 1981), which helped to explain what children were doing when they could participate in some parts of events and not others (e.g., "getting ready" routines). Reexamining the events that I had used in intervention, I realized that certain events emphasized some components over others, such as role relationships in restaurant events or action sequences in camping events. This was then incorporated into my theorizing about event representations and how to create meaningful intervention contexts. Finally, becoming acquainted with Gail Goodman's work allowed me to understand the process children go through as they form and use event representations. My journey illustrates how our intervention can become more theoretically motivated and how theories can become more sensitive using insights from clinical practice.

NOTE

I would like to thank the staff, children, and families of the Jowonio School, Syracuse, New York, who challenged me to develop an understanding of the importance of everyday events, not only for the use of language, but also to support successful participation in events. Special thanks go to Susan Gelling, Ellen Donovan, and Teri Paduana, who shared with me their insights as classroom teachers.

REFERENCES

Abelson, R. P. (1981). Psychological status of the script concept. *American Psychologist, 36* (7), 715–729.

Bruner, J. (1975). The ontogenesis of speech acts. *Journal of Child Language, 2,* 1–19.

Bruner, J., & Sherwood, V. (1976). Early rule structure: The case for peek-a-boo. In J. Bruner, A. Jolly, & K. Sylva (Eds.), *Play: Its role in evolution and development.* Harmondsworth, England: Penguin.

Constable, C. M. (1983). Creating communicative contexts. In H. Winitz (Ed.), *Language disorders: For clinicians, by clinicians.* Baltimore, MD: University Park Press.

Constable, C. M. (1986). The application of scripts in the organization of language intervention contexts. In K. Nelson (Ed.), *Event knowledge: Structure and function in development.* Hillsdale, NJ: Lawrence Erlbaum.

Culatta, B. (1984). A discourse-based approach to training grammatical rules. *Seminars in Speech and Language, 5,* 253–262.

DeMaio, L. J. (1984). Establishing communication networks through interactive play: A method for language programming in the clinic. *Seminars in Speech and Language, 5,* 199–210.

Duchan, J. F. (1991). Everyday events: Their role in language assessment and intervention. In T. M. Gallagher (Ed.), *Pragmatics of language: Clinical practice issues.* San Diego, CA: Singular Publishing Group.

Duchan, J., & Weitzner-Lin, B. (1987). Nurturant–naturalistic language intervention for language impaired children: Implications for planning lessons and tracking progress. *ASHA, 29,* 45–49.

Farrar, J., & Goodman, G. S. (1990). Developmental differences in the relation between scripts and episodic memory: Do they exist? In R. Fivush & J. Hudson (Eds.), *Knowing and remembering in young children* (pp. 30–64). New York: Cambridge University Press.

Farrar, J., & Goodman, G. S. (1992). Developmental changes in event memory. *Child Development, 63,* 173–187.

Fey, M. (1986). *Language intervention with young children.* San Diego, CA: College-Hill Press.

Kirchner, D. M. (1991). Reciprocal book reading: A discourse-based intervention strategy for the child with atypical language development. In T. M. Gallagher (Ed.), *Pragmatics of language: Clinical practice issues.* San Diego, CA: Singular Publishing Group.

Nelson, K. (1986). *Event knowledge: Structure and function in development.* Hillsdale, NJ: Lawrence Erlbaum.

Nelson, K., & Gruendel, J. (1979). At morning it's lunchtime: A scriptal view of children's dialogues. *Discourse Processes, 2,* 73–94.

Nelson, K., & Gruendel, J. (1981). Generalized event representations: Basic building blocks of cognitive development. In M. E. Lamb & A. L. Brown (Eds.), *Advances in developmental psychology* (Vol. 1, pp. 131–158). Hillsdale, NJ: Lawrence Erlbaum.

Ninio, A., & Bruner, J. (1978). The achievement and the antecedents of labeling. *Journal of Child Language, 5,* 1–15.

Price, D., & Goodman, G. S. (1990). Visiting the wizard: Children's memory for a recurring event. *Child Development, 61,* 664–680.

Ratner, N., & Bruner, J. (1978). Games, social exchange and the acquisition of language. *Journal of Child Language, 5,* 391–401.

Ross, B. L., & Berg, C. A. (1990). Individual differences in script reports: Implications for language assessment. *Topics in Language Disorders, 10,* 30–44.

Schank, R. C., & Abelson, R. P. (1977). *Scripts, plans, goals, and understanding.* Hillsdale, NJ: Lawrence Erlbaum.

Smith, B., Ratner, H. H., & Hobart, C. (1987). The role of cueing and organization in children's memory for events. *Journal of Experimental Child Psychology, 44,* 1–24.

Snyder-McLean, L. K., Solomonson, M. A., McLean, J. E., & Sack, S. (1984). Structuring joint action routines: A strategy for facilitating communication and language development in the classroom. *Seminars in Speech and Language, 5,* 213–225.

Weitzner-Lin, B., Sonnenmeier, R., & Murphy, D. (1983). *The use of formatted interactions in language intervention.* Paper presented at the Annual Convention of the American Speech Language and Hearing Association, Cincinnati, Ohio.

Westby, C. E. (1980). Assessment of cognitive and language abilities through play. *Language, Speech, and Hearing Services in Schools, 11,* 154–168.

Westby, C. E. (1988). Children's play: Reflections of social competence. *Seminars in Speech and Language, 9,* 1–13.

chapter 11

INTERVENTION PRINCIPLES FOR GESTALT-STYLE LEARNERS

Judith Felson Duchan

Most language intervention approaches are based on the assumption that the children learn by building from small to larger and more complex units (but for an exception, see Manning & Bobkoff Katz, 1989). This analytic bias also is fundamental to the conceptualization of pragmatically based intervention approaches. For example, **modeling techniques** elaborate on the form and content of what the child has just produced (Duchan & Weitzner-Lin, 1987; Girolametto, Greenberg, & Manolson, 1986), and **scaffolding approaches** provide the child with a fully scaffolded version of an event in hopes that the child will select individual elements and build them into a complete schema that they will use when experiencing that event (Kirchner, 1991; Snyder-McLean, Solomonson, McLean, & Sack, 1984).

The presumption of analytic intervention approaches is that gestalt units used by children are understood by them as analyzed composites. The children are seen as having created sentences and stories from the elements within them, as understanding the whole structure by building it up or processing it from its parts. However, there is considerable evidence from both normal and abnormal language learners that children (and adults, for that matter) sometimes understand what they hear, say, and do as unanalyzed gestalts, as whole memorized units rather than as an analyzed sum of their parts (Peters, 1983; Prizant, 1983; Wong-Fillmore, 1979). Indeed, some children have been found to favor this gestalt approach over an analytic one, as evidenced by their high frequency productions of (1) **single utterance routines**—phrases or clauses that are worded and expressed in the same way each time they are said (Peters, 1983; Prizant & Rydell, 1984; Wong-Fillmore, 1979); (2) **event routines**—activities that are produced in a preordained way, with little variation (Bruner, 1983; Farrar & Goodman, 1990; Kanner, 1943); and (3) **discourse routines**—strips of conversations, narratives, or television commercials that are memorized segments said with the same expressive elements and wording on repeated occasions (Anderson, Dunlea, & Kekelis, 1984; Bloom, 1970; Snow & Goldfield, 1983).

There are different renditions of gestalt learning and processing in the literature on language acquisition. Most commentators see the processing as normal and engaged in by all learners to different degrees (Peters, 1983; Prizant, 1983, Vihman, 1982; Wong-Fillmore, 1979). Where researchers and teachers are divided is on how to regard the children whose language is primarily comprised of gestalt forms to the exclusion of the analytic forms—the children characterized as having a "gestalt style" (e.g., Prizant, 1983).

One perspective on gestalt-style learning, a deficit view, holds that linguistic or conceptual gestalts are not productive, that children with gestalt styles are likely to be less proficient in their language than those who take an analytic approach to learning. The deficit view also assumes that any growth in language learning must be done analytically, and that linguistic gestalts be superseded by a second language system involving an analytic build-up approach. This view has been taken with regard to typical language learners learning a second language (Krashen & Scarcella, 1978) as well as atypical language learners learning their first language (Prizant, 1983; Prizant & Rydell, in press). The logical conclusion from the deficit view would be that language intervention should be designed to help gestalt learners develop an analytic approach to replace their gestalt one.

A second view takes gestalt-style learning as productive, creative, and legitimate. For example, Peters (1983), a proponent of this competence view, points to the natural occurrence of language routines in everyday language, such as those involved in greetings (how are you?), exclamations (oh boy), and social control (lookit, shut up). She sees these gestalts as efficient, in that they do not require re-creation with each use. Peters also suggests that the same language utterance can be represented as a gestalt and as component parts, and that routines often contain slots into which selected elements can be fit ("how are you"—completed by phrases such as "today, this morning, this evening"). The competence view, like the deficit view, is applied to typical children learning their first or second language (Peters, 1983; Wong-Fillmore, 1979) and to children diagnosed abnormal (e.g., blind children with gestalt styles; Landau & Gleitman, 1985; Urwin, 1979). The implication of this view is that language teachers or clinicians should let well enough alone and not institute language training to alter children's gestalt learning styles.

I suggest that a resolution of this issue of how to regard and treat gestalt learners should depend upon answers to questions such as the following:

1. Is the learner producing gestalts that contain elements that he or she is able to analyze on other occasions?
2. Are individual gestalts flexible, and if so, in what ways?
3. How do gestalts fit their contexts from the child's view and from the culturally conventional point of view?
4. How are individual gestalts structured and understood by the gestalt-style learner?
5. How do individual gestalts function for the gestalt-style learner?

I address these questions by examining various examples from the literature on typical language learners and from research on abnormal children who are autistic. I also draw from my own research on gestalt processing in a particular subject Aaron, a 20-year-old, who has been diagnosed autistic and whom my students and I have been studying (Duchan, 1991; Goldstein & Duchan, 1991; Sonnenmeier & Duchan, 1991). In the vein of recent theoretical articles on language intervention (Duchan, 1986; Johnston, 1985; Nelson, 1989), and in the tradition of Slobin (1973), I will frame my thoughts as intervention principles and associate a principle or two with each of the questions.

Question 1. Is the learner producing gestalts that contain elements that he or she is able to analyze on other occasions?

Language learning typically involves acquiring phrases or sayings such as "go for it" or "how are you." It has been hypothesized by Peters (1977, 1983) and others (e.g., Nagy, 1978) that these gestalt phrases are stored by adults as single linguistic entities, separate from their subparts, and that they can be analyzed into their constituents when the occasion calls for it (e.g., the producer of the phrases "go for it" and "how are you" might have to shift to analytic interpretation if they were to be received and responded to analytically as "I already went for it" or "I've been sick lately").

Peters's dual storage notion would suggest dividing gestalts into two types, those that the child analyzes in a second storage system, and those that are seen only as wholes. The intervention implication is to focus teaching on those gestalts whose elements are not stored elsewhere. The aim of the teaching would be to provide the child with a means for analyzing all gestalt forms.

But, unfortunately, the dual storage rendition of phrases will not account for everything that goes on in gestalt learning and processing. The dual storage, as described by Peters, is focused on phrases and does not consider events-gestalts or long unanalyzed segments of discourse. Also, some gestalts cannot be rendered as productive forms when analyzed, such as the impenetrable gestalts from a second language (e.g., oy vey iz mir, by someone who does not understand Yiddish) or ditties from an unknown historical past (Ring around the Rosy). Further, there are gestalts that are partially but not fully analyzed as they are produced, such as ones that have open slots for additions (a ritualized school activity on calendars involving day and date changes).

Nonetheless, we can arrive at intervention principles for handling gestalts that exclude event and discourse routines and impenetrable utterance routines. The principles rest on the results of evaluating a learner's individual gestalts to determine whether they are dually stored, and if not whether the child may benefit by learning to understand the gestalt analytically.

Wong-Fillmore (1979) provides an example of gestalts stored only as gestalts and not as analyzed elements. She found that Spanish-speaking children when first learning English learned single-utterance gestalts, rather than individual words. The expressions served a variety of functions: to create an appearance of understanding (Oh Yeah? Hey, what's going on here?); to participate in repeating activities (Me first. No fair); and to request information (What's happening? I don't understand). Wong-Fillmore commented that these students had little understanding of the semantics or syntax of these utterance routines, as was indicated by their lack of display of such understanding in their analytic language. Helping these children analyze the elements of their unanalyzed gestalts would be a worthwhile teaching endeavor.

Examples of dually stored gestalts can also be found in the productions of gestalt learners. Our subject Aaron used a number of utterance routines that were not only related to the situation but were also within his semantic and syntactic capability. For example, he said "Put that pizza down" as a pizza was being ordered and throughout the time he waited for it. The phrase was often accompanied by a hand gesture from mouth to table, as if putting a piece of pizza down from his mouth to a plate. Phrases such as these qualified as gestalts in that they were said with the same intonation and wording, did not follow the conversational flow, and were copies of what he had heard and said previously. However, these gestalts were analyzed, as evidenced by the fact that they contained lexical items related to the ongoing situation, the semantic and syntactic components were productive for him on other occasions, and he was able to answer questions put to him about the utterances. For Aaron, remediation which would be aimed at teaching him the elements of these gestalt forms would have been redundant and therefore inappropriate.

These two examples lead to two related intervention principles:

Intervention Principle 1A: If the learner does not know the elements of a gestalt, consider the usefulness of helping the child understand its elements. If deemed useful, help the child analyze the gestalt.

Intervention Principle 1B: If the learner knows the elements of a gestalt, do not work on teaching them.

A second question, related to the first, is the following:

Question 2. Are individual gestalts flexible, and if so, in what ways?

Katherine Nelson has depicted typically developing children in their earliest years as conceiving of events such as daily routines as gestalts, as "conceptual wholes," whose "constituent parts—objects—are not at first salient referents for the words being learned" (Nelson, 1991, p. 105). Bates and her colleagues also describe children as using unanalyzed gestalts at this early stage (Bates, Bretherton, Shore, & McNew, 1983). They describe the processing of events as involving an activation of all the links in the event at once. In this preverbal stage "the child does not yet actively select portions of this knowledge to stand for or remind him of other elements" (p. 110). The researchers propose that the child moves from gestalt to analytic conceptualizations through slot learning, wherein various elements are inserted into a slot in the gestalt and the children learn about syntagmatic relationships by coming to understand where the slots are, and paradigmatic categories by understanding what sorts of elements fit in the slots. A game of catch involves different balls, a birthday party, different presents. Thus it is that children are seen to develop an analytic understanding of the components of the routine.

Aaron's routines varied from one another in their degree of flexibility. Some were rendered as exact duplicates whenever they were performed; others varied considerably on different occasions. An example of the invariant routines was a story, performed three times, which Aaron titled "Wanda the Witch." Each performance involved a lengthy enactment of a Sesame Street poem containing multiple examples of the letter W. Aaron's depiction of the poem on each occasion included the same voice changes, dialect shifts (from American to British accents), exaggerated chanting of particular lines, and hand movements marking the regularities in rhythm. Interruptions that occurred during the performance were ignored, and most questions about the story were answered incorrectly. The constellation of evidence would suggest that this particular routine was stored as a vivid gestalt, an inflexible one.

The inflexibility of Wanda the Witch can be contrasted with the highly flexible gestalt that Aaron called the "more or less poem." This poem was performed by Aaron at the beginning of a two-hour pizza party. He asked: "Do more or less poem?" and when granted permission carried out an animated performance before an audience, and in front of a mirror. It began as follows:

Once there was one more.
and then there were [#] more.
and more (high-pitched voice).
and again mwah mwah mwah mwah mwah mwah mwah mwah.
(sung, ranging from low- to high-pitched voice.)
now there are less.

The phrase "more or less" contained in the poem became a theme phrase throughout the two-hour period. It grew and changed as it incorporated information about what was going on and combined with other rhythmic single-utterances routines. So, pizza became part of the "more or less" phrase when pizza was ordered, grape juice during and after the time grape juice was being made, and mention of aspects of the videotaping occurred throughout. Examples of Aaron's flexibility can be seen below:

> More and less pizza then do more and less poem.
> More or less grape juice poem for dinner.
> More or less pizza poem.
> Aaron do the more pizza poem.
> Do camera, more pizza and grape juice poem.
> More or less pizza on the video camera.
> More or less pizza poem grape juice poem.
> More or less pizza poem on the vcr.
> More or less grape juice pizza poem.
> Ernie and Bert's more less pizza.
> More or less poem on the tenth of September.

What seems to govern Aaron's creations of phrases and their combinations are the rhythmic alternations produced by strong and weak syllables. In many of the one-liners one finds duplicates of a five-beat rhythmic pattern: strong (/), two weaks (UU), a second strong (/), and a final optional weak ((U)): (/UU/(U)).

> more or less poem (/UU/U)
> more or less pizza (/UU/U)
> video camera (/UU/U)
> tenth of September (/UU/U)
> more or less grape juice (/UU/U)
> poem for dinner (/UU/U)
> Ernie and Bert (/UU/)

In Aaron's case, we would not recommend working with him to analyze the Wanda the Witch story, but rather allow him to perform it to appreciative audiences and not to perform it in contexts where it is at cross purposes with the ongoing event (e.g., conversations, on the job).

Aaron's flexible utterance and discourse gestalts adhered to a rhythmic structuring, at the expense of semantics and syntax, resulting in cryptic and unconventional phrases such as "More or less poem on the tenth of September." A potential approach would be to allow him his rhythmic structuring but challenge him to be more contextually relevant in his selection of lexical items for building his poetic gestalts (I'd like some pizza; I made the grape juice). These suggestions for handling Aaron's routines fit the following intervention principles:

Intervention Principle 2A: For gestalts that are inflexible, ignore them or disallow them in contexts where they are interfering.

Intervention Principle 2B: For those that are flexible determine their dimensions of flexibility and expand on them.

So far we have been discussing the internal structure of individual gestalts. A third factor affecting the way gestalts are used has to do with how they are associated with the particular situational events. This leads to a third question:

Question 3. How do gestalts fit their contexts from the child's view and from the culturally conventional point of view?

It is not always easy to tell how routines fit the ongoing context. A naive observer would assume that a child saying "Don't throw the dog off the balcony" when he was pushing a cup off a table was not talking about anything in the current here and now. However the child producing that well-known phrase (see Kanner, 1943; 1946) seemed to be using it in contexts in which he was about to violate a rule. The phrase originated several years earlier when he was about to throw a toy animal from a balcony and was told not to. He seemed to be using the phrase in contexts where he was doing something wrong.

Researchers in the deficit frame have assumed that routines that do not make conventional sense are unrelated to the context. The routines are often called "empty" or "rote," indicating an assumption that they are lacking in not only semantic or syntactic content, but also intentional or situational meaning.

Those taking a competence view would assume that gestalt forms have relevance for the child, and that they probably bear some relationship to the current context. The relationship may be unconventional, as when language forms are not interpretable in light of what is taking place, as in the case of "Don't throw the dog off the balcony"; or it may be conventionally interpretable, as in Wong-Fillmore's examples of "Me first," "No fair," and "What's happening?"

Our subject, Aaron, used both unconventionally and conventionally contextualized routines. Examples of his unconventional routines were a group of three, which he used to indicate the beginning or ending of events. He enacted the beginning song from the Electric Company to start events ("We're gonna turn it on, we're gonna turn on the power") and both Sesame Street and Electric Company credits to say goodbye to people as they left the event ("Sesame Street is a production of the Children's Television Workshop. Bye

Holly"). His more conventional routines were those that served to manage the discourse of the interaction. Examples are "Wait a minute, please," "Excuse me, please," and "Whatever they are."

Each of Aaron's routine types calls for a different intervention. The conventional routines can be left alone. For the unconventional ones, he might be encouraged to substitute more conventional sayings such as "See you later alligator" rather than "Sesame Street is a production of the Children's Television Workshop." These examples can be expressed in intervention principles as follows:

> **Intervention Principle 3A: If a gestalt form is *unconventionally contextualized,* work on teaching a conventional routine or analyzed unit that would fit the context better.**

> **Intervention Principle 3B: If the form is *conventionally contextualized,* but not analyzed by the child, work on teaching how to build on the relationship between the form and situational context and generalizing this understanding to other situations.**

Until now we have been considering whether gestalts can be analyzed, whether they are used in flexible ways, and how they fit their context. We now move to a fourth question, which asks not only about the degree of structure, flexibility, and conventionality, but what it is that seems to be holding the gestalt together as a gestalt form.

> **Question 4. How are individual gestalts structured and understood by the gestalt-style learner?**

Studies of gestalt structuring have been done in the tradition of conventional linguistics, which emphasizes semantic and syntactic analysis. This linguistic analytically based research approach best fits the analytic learner, who builds up meanings and syntax from individual- to multiple-word utterances. But what is going on for the child who does not approach language in that way? There is a second, less emphasized literature in the area of child language that focuses more on the poetic nature of language expression than its linguistic structure.

Older children have been found to produce poetic stories, which cohere not only linguistically, but also rhythmically, intonationally, or thematically as gestalts. Gee (1991), in his study of a seven-year-old child who tells stories in the style of her African-American cultural tradition, describes her as follows: "She uses a good deal of syntactic parallelism, repetition, and sound devices (phonological sequences, intonation and rate changes) to set up rhythmic and poetic patterning within and across her stanzas" (p. 10). Sutton-Smith (1986) finds that poetic stories are told by many young children, not just those whose adult culture has the forms: "The children raise the pitch of their voices, they give a slower delivery, there is more word emphasis, there may be exaggerated sounds, there is a regular beat to the telling of the story which tends to come in regular lines as in verse, and they may give a rhythmic delivery and use dramatic crescendos" (p.75).

These poetic gestalts are also formed by abnormal children. For example, Prizant and Rydell describe a subject who played with one of his gestalt expressions as follows: "one child repeated 'it's a piece of sponge' over 40 times in rapid succession including changes in stress patterns and intonation" (Prizant & Rydell, 1984, p. 190).

Our subject Aaron's utterance, event, and discourse routines were rich in poetic elements. Some of the routines were sung and danced; many included a wide assortment of voice changes, a variety of repeating rhythms, and intricate patterns of rhyme and alliteration.

The literature on expressive, poetic language suggests that some of Aaron's routines may be elaborately organized as poems. Interventions that treat the gestalt as solely analyzable into syntactic or semantic components may be missing an important side of what the child is attempting to do. Evidence for such a mismatch between a child's attempt to form a poetic gestalt and a linguistically based response to it is found in the experience of Deena, a kindergartner studied by Sara Michaels (Michaels, 1986). Deena's sharing-time event descriptions were complex poetic constructions. Her teacher, who was looking for logical single-topic descriptions, regarded Deena's poems as wandering attempts to describe an event. Deena was aware of the teacher's disfavor and described her teacher as never allowing her to finish (Michaels & Cazden, 1986).

Before instituting intervention that will help children analyze their gestalt forms, the teacher or clinician needs to determine how the gestalts are structured. This claim can be formed as the following intervention principle:

Intervention Principle 4: Base intervention on how the learner organizes the gestalt and assigns it meaning. If the gestalt routines are composites of expressive elements, do not force them to be analyzed into semantic or syntactic components that may have little relevance in their construction.

Our next and last question pushes the previous four (which focus mostly on the structure and meaning) into the domain of function by asking:

Question 5. How do individual gestalts function for the gestalt-style learner?

Peters (1977, 1983), in an effort to determine why some normally developing children use a gestalt learning style, speculates that the gestalt learners use language most often to achieve social goals, whereas the analytic learners are more interested in using language to gain information about the world.

Peters's evidence for her social function hypothesis is drawn from the work of Katherine Nelson (1973), who differentiated language learners into two types: expressive and referential. The expressive children (Peters calls them gestalt learners) often used personal–social phrases as their first productions, phrases expressing feelings, needs, and social niceties (e.g., go away, stop it, don't do it, thank you, I want it). The referential children during their early stages of language production used mostly single nouns and used them to refer to objects or events.

Peters argues that their different communicative goals lead them to tune in to different elements of their environmental language. The elements that the expressive children pick up are those that they hear used by the adults to manage social interaction, the very phrases that qualify as gestalt forms under Peters's criteria.

The social function theory of Peters, when extended, could imply that all gestalt forms are aimed at achieving social functions. This is not the case, as is indicated by the discovery of gestalts that are self-directed rather than socially directed (e.g., Prizant & Rydell, 1984, in press; and Aaron's soliloquies, see previous discussion). Many routinized forms are performed when the learner is alone and appear to be for pleasure or aimed at practicing or regulating behavior or as expressions of emotional content.

A self-directed routine should be regarded and treated differently from a social one. A self-directed routine may be carried out quietly, and in the privacy of one's own place, while a social one, by definition, requires the interaction of another. The broader principle is that intervention techniques used with gestalt learners should vary depending upon how particular gestalts are used.

Simons (1974) follows this notion of tailoring intervention to a function. For example, she uses a "cutting through" approach with children who are aware of their routine and are using it to "manipulate the environment." She describes the effect of cutting through for Jack, a six-year-old who felt compelled to "march up and down the stairs in a straight line like a soldier, turn back, proceed to the bathroom and start screaming on his way" (pp. 7–8). Simons noted that the child did this only when others were on the stairs. She talked with the child about his compulsion (cut through it) and allowed him to carry out his action only when others were not on the stairs. The child immediately abandoned the activity.

Our subject Aaron used different routines to achieve different communicative goals. He effectively used them to greet, say goodbye, entertain, avoid responding, reprimand himself, and manage social interactions. The fact that Aaron was able to achieve his goals suggests that the routines be let alone. But because they were unconventional and difficult to interpret by those who do not know him, he might be provided with some alternative forms, more conventional ones, so that he can still achieve his communicative goal.

Intervention Principle 5: Analyze each gestalt for its function, and design the intervention approach to be in accord with what the learner is trying to accomplish with the gestalt.

*   *   *

This chapter, framed around five questions, offered intervention principles to guide one's thinking and tactics for interacting with gestalt-style learners. The aim was to develop a competence view of the gestalt-style learner. The approach was to examine the gestalts produced by the child in order to determine whether or not the child understands their semantic or syntactic make up, the degree to which the gestalts were flexible, how (or whether) the child relates the gestalts to the current situation, how the child constructs particular gestalts, and what function those gestalts serve.

Answers to the questions lead to different intervention approaches. The implications of the findings are that some gestalt expressions should be encouraged, others be made more conventional, and still others should be eliminated and a substitute created to achieve their function.

An underlying assumption of some of the principles is that children should be taught to analyze their own gestalt productions. Such an analytic approach would allow them to learn the elements, and how they combine. Evidence that this approach is potentially effective comes from the acquisition literature on typical and atypical gestalt learners who use open slots in gestalts to arrive at analytic categories and who practice breaking down gestalt utterances to discover their elements (Baltaxe & Simmons, 1977; Clark, 1974; Wong-Fillmore, 1979). These two methods, that of **slot filling** and **breaking down gestalt units,** are appropriate when the children have not learned to analyze particular gestalts, yet use them appropriately in the context (e.g., wait a minute, me first, no fair). They might help the child who is committed to gestalts governed by events by providing him or her a more flexible version of the gestalt, one that is analyzable into varying poetic, meaning, or linguistic elements.

Analyzing gestalts is less useful when the gestalts are not conventionally related to the context (Don't throw the dog off the balcony), or when they are organized using a poetic rather than a linguistic base (e.g., more or less poem on the tenth of September). In these cases the best approach may be to respond to the gestalt according to how it appears to be understood by the gestalt user, and then to offer a substitute or respond in kind if the situation allows for it. Rather than chastising the child about the inappropriateness of saying something about dogs and balconies when they are not present, the interactant might respond "you'd better not!" as the child announces a wrongdoing. Or "I'm doing something wrong" could be modelled so as to provide the child with a more conventional substitute phrase. Similarly, rather than taking issue with Aaron for uttering what seems to be nonsense, the interactant might respond with yet another rhythm to fit Aaron's. This was Oliver

Sacks's approach when he provided eight-digit prime numbers (numbers that could be divided by no other whole number except itself, or one) to twin savants who enjoyed creating up to six-digit prime numbers for each other (Sacks, 1970). This tack of **joining in** the interest of the other could also help that other person build more conventional forms, if the expression used in joining in creates an interactive context that extends beyond or is more conventional than that existing in the original context.

To conclude, the analytic approaches to language intervention are likely to ignore the importance of gestalt learning in the development of communication in both normal and abnormal gestalt learners. With the insights from pragmatics that have led us to focus on larger gestalt units such as routinized utterances, events, and discourse units, we can begin to tailor our intervention approaches to the particular ways learners understand and use gestalt forms.

REFERENCES

Anderson, E., Dunlea, A., & Kekelis, L. (1984). Blind children's language: Resolving some differences. *Journal of Child Language, 11,* 645–664.

Baltaxe, C., & Simmons, J. (1977). Bedtime soliloquies and linguistic competence in autism. *Journal of Speech and Hearing Disorders, 42,* 376–393.

Bates, E., Bretherton, I., Shore, C., & McNew, S. (1983). Names, gestures, & objects: The role of context in the emergence of symbols. In K. Nelson (Ed.), *Children's language* (Vol 4, pp. 59–123). Hillsdale, NJ: Lawrence Erlbaum.

Bloom, L. (1970). *Language development: Form and function in emerging grammars.* Cambridge MA: The M.I.T. Press.

Brown, R., & Hanlon, C. (1970). Derivational complexity and order of acquisition in child speech. In J. Hayes (Ed.), *Cognition and the development of language* (pp. 155–207). New York: Wiley.

Bruner, J. (1983). *Child's talk: Learning to use language.* New York: W. W. Norton.

Clark, R. (1974). Performing without competence. *Journal of Child Language, 1,* 1–10.

Duchan, J. (1986). Language intervention through sensemaking and fine tuning. In R. Schiefelbusch (Ed.), *Language competence: Assessment and intervention* (pp. 182–212). San Diego, CA: College-Hill Press.

Duchan, J. (1991). Everyday events: Their role in language assessment and intervention. In T. Gallagher (Ed.), *Pragmatics of language: Clinical practice issues* (pp. 43–98). San Diego, CA: Singular Publishing Group.

Duchan, J., & Weitzner-Lin, B. (1987). Nuturant-naturalistic intervention for language-impaired children: Implications for planning lessons and tracking progress. *ASHA, 29,* 45–49.

Farrar, M., & Goodman, G. (1990). Developmental differences in the relation between episodic and semantic memory. Do they exist? In R. Fivush & J. Hudson (Eds.), *Knowing and remembering in young children* (pp. 33–64). New York: Cambridge University Press.

Gee, J. (1991). Memory and myth: A perspective on narrative. In A. McCabe & C. Peterson (Eds.), *Developing narrative structure* (pp. 1–25). Hillsdale, NJ: Lawrence Erlbaum.

Girolometto, L., Greenberg, J., & Manolson, A. (1986). Developing dialogue skills: The Hanen early language parent program. *Seminars in Speech and Language, 7,* 367–382.

Goldstein, K., & Duchan, J. (1991). *Interactions with and without routines by an autistic young adult.* Paper presented at New York State Speech, Language, and Hearing Association Convention, Monticello, New York.

Johnston, J. (1985). Fit, focus and functionality: An essay on early language intervention. *Child Language Teaching and Therapy, 1,* 125–134.

Kanner, L. (1943). Autistic disturbances of affective contact. *Nervous Child, 2,* 217–250.

Kanner, L. (1946). Irrelevant and metaphorical language in early infantile autism. *American Journal of Psychiatry, 103,* 242–245.

Kirchner, D. (1991). Reciprocal book reading: A discourse-based intervention strategy for the child with atypical language development. In T. Gallagher (Ed.), *Pragmatics of language: Clinical practice issues* (pp. 307–332). San Diego, CA: Singular Publishing Group.

Krashen, S., & Scarcella, R. (1978). On routines and patterns in language acquisition and performance. *Language Learning, 28,* 283–300.

Landau, B., & Gleitman, L. (1985). *Language and experience: Evidence from the blind child.* Cambridge, MA: Harvard University Press.

Manning, A., & Bobkoff Katz, D. (1989). Language-learning patterns in echolalic children. *Child Language Teaching and Therapy, 5,* 249–261.

Michaels, S. (1986). Narrative presentations: An oral preparation for literacy with first graders. In J. Cook-Gumperz (Ed.), *The social construction of literacy* (pp. 91–116). New York: Cambridge University Press, 1986.

Michaels, S., & Cazden, C. (1986). Teacher–child collaboration as oral preparation for literacy. In B. Schieffelin & P. Gilmore (Eds.), *The acquisition of literacy: Ethnographic perspectives.* Norwood, NJ: Ablex Publishing.

Nagy, W. (1978). Some non-idiom larger-than-word units in the lexicon. *Papers from the Parasession on the Lexicon* (pp. 289–300). Chicago: Chicago Linguistics Society.

Nelson, K. (1973). Structure and strategy in learning how to talk. *Monographs of the Society for Research in Child Development, 38* (149).

Nelson, K. (1991). Concepts and meaning in language development. In N. Krasnegor, D. Rumbaugh, R. Schiefelbusch, & M. Studdert-Kennedy (Eds.), *Biological and behavioral determinants of language development* (pp. 89–115). Hillsdale, NJ: Lawrence Erlbaum.

Nelson, K. E. (1989). Strategies for first language teaching. In M. Rice & R. Schiefelbusch (Eds.), *The teachability of language* (pp. 263–310). Baltimore, MD: Paul H. Brookes.

Peters, A. (1977). Language learning strategies: Does the whole equal the sum of the parts? *Language, 53,* 560–573.

Peters, A. (1983). *The units of language acquisition.* New York: Cambridge University Press.

Prizant, B. (1983). Language acquisition and the communicative behavior in autism: Toward an understanding of the "whole" of it. *Journal of Speech and Hearing Disorders, 48,* 296–307.

Prizant, B., & Rydell, P. (1984). Analysis of functions of delayed echolalia in autistic children. *Journal of Speech and Hearing Research, 27,* 183–192.

Prizant, B., & Rydell, P. (in press). Assessment and intervention considerations for unconventional verbal behavior. In J. Reichle & D. Wacker (Eds.). *Communicative approaches to the management of challenging behavior.* Baltimore, MD: Paul H. Brookes.

Sacks, O. (1970). *The man who mistook his wife for a hat.* New York: Harper.

Simons, J. (1974). Observations on compulsive behavior in autism. *Journal of Autism and Childhood Schizophrenia, 4,* 1–10.

Slobin, D. (1973). Cognitive prerequisites for the acquisition of grammar. In C. Ferguson & D. Slobin (Eds.), *Studies of child language development.* New York: Holt, Rinehart and Winston.

Snow C., & Goldfield, B. (1983). Turn the page please: Situation-specific language learning. *Journal of Child Language, 10,* 551–570.

Snyder-McLean, L., Solomonson, B., McLean, J., & Sack, S. (1984). Structuring joint action routines: A strategy for facilitating communication and language development in the classroom. *Seminars in Speech and Language, 5,* 213–228.

Sonnenmeier, R., & Duchan, J. (1991). *Routinized verbal exchanges with autistic teenagers.* Miniseminar presentation at the American Speech-Language-Hearing Association, Annual Convention, Atlanta, Georgia.

Sutton-Smith, B. (1986). Children's fiction making. In T. Sarbin (Ed.), *Narrative psychology: The storied nature of human conduct.* New York: Praeger.

Urwin, C. (1979). Preverbal communication and early language development in blind children. *Papers and Reports on Child Language Development, 17,* 119–127. Stanford, CA: Department of Linguistics, Stanford University.

Urwin, C. (1983). Dialogue and cognitive functioning in the early language development of three blind children. In A. Mills (Ed.), *Language acquisition in the blind child: Normal and deficient* (pp. 142–161). San Diego, CA: College-Hill Press.

Vihman, M. (1982). Formulas in first and second language acquisition. In L. Obler & L. Menn (Eds.), *Exceptional language and linguistics* (pp. 261–284). New York: Academic Press.

Wong-Fillmore, L. (1979). Individual differences in second language acquisition. In C. Fillmore, D. Kempler, & W. Wang (Eds.), *Individual differences in language ability and language behavior.* New York: Academic Press.

APPENDIX AND SUMMARY

How We Might Go About Establishing Intervention Goals for Gestalt-Style Learners: Guiding Questions and Principles

Q1. Is the learner producing gestalts that contain elements that he or she is able to analyze on other occasions?

> P1A: If the learner does not know the elements of a gestalt, consider the usefulness of helping the child understand its elements. If deemed useful, help the child analyze the gestalt.

> P1B: If the learner knows the elements of a gestalt, do not work on teaching them.

Q2. Are individual gestalts flexible, and if so, in what ways?

> P2A: For gestalts that are inflexible, ignore them or disallow them in contexts where they are interfering.

> P2B: For those that are flexible determine their dimensions of flexibility and expand on them.

Q3. How do gestalts fit their contexts from the child's view and from the culturally conventional point of view?

> P3A: If a gestalt form is *unconventionally contextualized,* work on teaching a conventional routine or analyzed unit that would fit the context better.

> P3B: If the form is *conventionally contextualized,* but not analyzed by the child, work on teaching how to build on the realtionship between the form and situational context and generalizing this understanding to other situations.

Q4. How are individual gestalts structured and understood by the gestalt-style learner?

> P4: Base intervention on how the learner organizes the gestalt and assigns it meaning. If the gestalt routines are composites of expressive elements, do not force them to be analyzed into semantic or syntactic components that may have little relevance in their construction.

Q5. How do individual gestalts function for the gestalt-style learner?

> P5: Analyze each gestalt for its function, and design the intervention approach to be in accord with what the learner is trying to accomplish with the gestalt.

chapter 12

WHAT IS SO HARD ABOUT LEARNING TO READ?
A Pragmatic Analysis
Catherine E. Snow

Most children learn to talk relatively easily and quickly; often these same children have considerable difficulty learning to read. The question that is addressed in this chapter is: Why is it so much harder to learn to read than to learn to talk? Children learn language, in most cases, with only the help of untrained tutors—parents and older siblings; in order to learn to read most of them require the aid of highly trained teachers with special degrees in early childhood education. Children typically have learned most of what they need to know to use oral language effectively by age three or four, whereas most don't even start to try to figure out how to read till age five or six. Furthermore, the incidence of problems in acquiring language is smaller than the incidence of reading problems.

At the bare minimum it would seem that learning to read should be no harder than learning to talk. After all, language is closely related to reading, both theoretically (reading is, in some sense, oral language written down) and empirically (indicators of oral language skill predict reading ability fairly closely, and conversely children who have problems with oral language typically also have difficulty in acquiring literacy). In fact, as an abstract system reading should be considerably **easier** to acquire than oral language, if only because learners can build upon all they already know of language. So what is so hard about learning to read?

TABLE 12-1   Domains of Language and Literacy Skills

DOMAIN	MANIFESTATION IN LANGUAGE	SKILL ADDED FOR USE IN LITERACY
Phonology	Rules for sounds, sound sequences	Segmentation, abstraction of underlying forms
Grammar	Rules governing correctness of sentences	Literacy-specific grammatical constructions
Lexicon	Words encountered and used orally	Greatly expanded repertoire
Speech acts	Expressing communicative intents appropriately	Understanding communicative intent of literacy
Conversation	Rules for turn taking, face-to-face exchange	Avoiding pragmatics of face-to-face exchange
Connected discourse	Rules for making links across utterances	Constraints of distanced discourse and audience

I will attempt to answer this question by explicating the aspects of the language system that are relevant to reading acquisition, and for each aspect pointing out what it is that children have to add or to change in order to master literacy. In other words, given a five- or six-year-old child who controls the oral language system to an age-appropriate degree, what else must that child learn in order to become literate?

Considerable thinking and research have been done on some of the domains in which literacy makes demands that go beyond those of oral language. In particular, much attention has been paid to the role of metalinguistic and segmentation skills as prerequisites to early reading development. I will review research about these domains briefly in the following discussion; a more extensive discussion of the relevant literature can be found in Snow and Tabors (in press). I will argue, though, that much of the additional learning children must do to become literate relates not to phonological or grammatical analysis, but to pragmatics. I will show that the pragmatics of language use in literate and oral contexts differ very severely, but that children may approach literacy without realizing the impact of these differences. Children who assume that the pragmatic system they rely upon in oral language will serve them as well for reading may encounter serious problems in the acquisition of literacy.

THE LANGUAGE SYSTEM

Let us start, then, with a brief review of what the five-year-old already knows about language. Language skills can be analyzed for our purposes into six components, domains, or rule systems (Table 12-1): phonology, grammar, lexicon, speech acts, conversation, and connected discourse. Because this is a somewhat unconventional way of compartmentalizing language knowledge, it perhaps makes sense to present the criteria I use to define these domains. I take as a separate domain a component of language knowledge that has its own rule system referring to entities not referred to in the other rule systems and that has rules that are sufficiently language-specific that they vary across languages or language communities.

For example, the rules of phonology and grammar govern the production of forms that are correct and interpretable. Phonology deals with the sounds of words, and grammar with the forms of words and of sentences. Phonological rules refer to units such as phonemes, morphological boundaries, word boundaries, and syllables; grammatical rules operate on units that consist of sentence constituents (e.g., noun phrase, sentence subject), word classes (e.g., noun, preposition), and morphemes. The rules identify sequences that are acceptable and prescribe relationships between structure and interpretation.

Lexicon refers to the component of the langue system more generally referred to as vocabulary—the words one knows. The lexicon stores information about both word meaning and correct contexts of word use. Information about syntactic frames within which words can appear must be stored in the lexicon, as is information about how words are related to one another, both paradigmatically and syntagmatically.

The rule system for expressing communicative intents effectively and appropriately refers to units of analysis like speech acts and interactive contexts and to variables like social distance, relative power, degree of face threat, and situational informality. No one has, of course, fully formulated the rules for being effective and appropriate in expressing communicative intents, any more than anyone has fully explicated the rules of grammar or phonology for any language, but theoretical discussions like those of Austin (1962), Searle (1969), Ninio and Snow (1988), Dore (1974, 1975), and Brown and Levinson (1978) have at least identified the variables of importance and have started to hint at what the rules would look like.

Communicative intents as a domain are distinct from conversation as a domain, because the unit of analysis to which conversational rules apply is the turn, not the speech act, and because conversational rules govern participation in linguistic exchanges, not effectiveness of expressing communicative intent. Thus, preverbal children whose babbles, smiles, and gestures are timed to begin as their mothers' utterances end can be said to have mastered some of the rules of conversational turn taking, quite independent of their capacity to express specific communicative intents. To participate in more sophisticated conversations, one must also control the local rules for appropriate inter-turn pauses, distinguish an interruption from a back-channel, identify turns to which responses are obligatory, and in many other ways understand the local system governing the exchange of talk.

Finally, rules for connected discourse specify relations across utterance or sentence boundaries. It is perhaps valuable to contrast explicitly the rules of grammar and those governing connected discourse. Connected discourse rules enable speakers to make explicit relations between utterances, whereas grammatical rules operate within sentences. Examples of rules governing production and interpretation of connected discourse include the following: rules for the interpretation of pronouns or of definite noun phrases whose referents have been introduced earlier in the discourse; rules for interpreting sentence-linking forms like "afterwards," "meanwhile," "nonetheless," and "however", or rules for interpreting aspect and tense within narratives as signals of foregrounded versus backgrounded information. The units of analysis within which rules of connected discourse operate are texts rather than sentences, utterances, turns, or words.

As can be seen in Table 12–1, these six domains of languge are all characterized by their own units of analysis and their own sets of relevant variables. They also show characteristic developmental courses and seem to be characterized by differing degrees of reliance on or vulnerability to environmental factors during development. Most important for our current discussion, though, they all relate to the demands of literacy in somewhat different ways.

LANGUAGE-LITERACY RELATIONSHIPS IN FAMILIAR DOMAINS

Phonology in Oral Language and Literacy

For children who need to learn to read an alphabetic language, it is clear that one obstacle is identifying the units represented by letters. As Liberman, Shankweiler, Liberman, Fowler, and Fischer pointed out in 1977, the sounds represented by most consonants are unpronounceable in isolation. Children must come to understand that the letter "b" stands for an abstract entity, not for the syllable "buh," for example. Understanding that spoken syllables and words can be segmented into smaller units and divining the crucial characteristics of those units are difficult tasks that must be at least initiated before alphabetic reading can make any sense.

Evidence suggesting that phonological segmentation skills must be added to the phonological system if children are to become literate derives from studies showing that children who are better at rhyming, at deleting initial or final sounds from words, and at invented spelling, learn to read more easily (Bradley & Bryant, 1985; Helfgott, 1976; Read, 1975, 1986; Treiman & Baron, 1981; Vellutino & Scallon, 1987). However, there is also evidence that children get to be better at phonemic segmentation skills as they get to be better readers, which of course makes perfect sense since exposure to the spelling system is one source of solid information about possible segmentations (Ehri, 1984).

Grammar in Oral and Written Language

We know that certain complex grammatical structures are much more common in written than in oral forms. Oral English produced on line is characterized by a high proportion of animate and pronominal subjects, and by heavily right-branching structures. In written language "heavy" subjects (full noun phrases, noun phrases modified by adjectives or relatives, or sentential structures) are much more common, as are left-branching or embedded structures. Producing such literate sentences requires considerably more planning time and energy than does producing typically "oral" sentences, and comprehending them certainly requires extra effort (as anyone who has listened to a written paper read aloud knows all too well).

Poor readers often show deficits in grammatical processing skills (Mann, 1991) and in tasks reflecting awareness of grammatical rules (Ryan & Ledger, 1984). Such deficits may relate to general language processing problems that also cause difficulties in learning to read, or may conversely reflect lack of exposure to the grammatical forms encountered in literate contexts.

Vocabulary

The vast majority of the vocabulary items any adult knows have been encountered primarily in literate contexts. When children start to learn to read, their texts are typically constrained to the three or four thousand most common vocabulary items—all of which the child is likely to know and use in oral contexts (Hayes & Ahrens, 1988). However, by about grade four children are encountering many less frequent lexical items in the texts they are expected to read. Children with small oral vocabularies may be reading many words they do not know or use orally. They need somehow to expand their vocabularies in order to understand texts that contain these words; paradoxically, the best way to expand their vocabularies is to acquire them in context from understanding the texts within which the new words are encountered (Adams, 1990).

LANGUAGE-LITERACY RELATIONSHIPS
IN PRAGMATIC DOMAINS

I will argue that the three domains of language competence that are traditionally grouped together under the rubric "pragmatics" are the site of the greatest differences between oral and written language. Essentially, I will suggest that the pragmatics of face-to-face communication are seductive and are assumed by children and even sometimes by adults to define the only pragmatic demands of communication. However, the task of meeting pragmatic demands can be much greater in written than in oral communication, and some of the specific mechanisms that have been developed for meeting those demands in literate contexts are quite different from the mechanisms we use during oral, face-to-face communication.

Pragmatics is defined as the systems of rules designed to ensure that language use is interpersonally appropriate and that it is effective in ensuring that the speaker's or author's intent is understood. Thus, for example, pragmatics encompasses the rules for the polite and effective expression of speech acts, the appropriate exchange of conversational turns, and the interpretable linking of utterances to one another in a larger discourse. Pragmatics also encompasses rules governing the expression and interpretation of the speaker's perspective on what is being expressed, and rules for suggesting what the listener's perspective should be.

We will discuss the differences between oral and literate pragmatics in three subdomains: expressing speech acts, regulating conversational exchange, and making connections across utterances in larger discourse units.

Speech Acts

Children acquire language in order to have an effect on the world—to express their own intentions and get others to listen and respond to those intentions. Young children seem to be rather precocious in speech act development—differentiating many different categories of speech acts from one another, for example—compared at least to their grammatical or lexical development.

Of course, people write in order to have an effect on the world too—to argue, convince, entertain, and so on. But most children are exposed to literacy first through reading, not through writing, and it is not always unambiguous to young children what the pragmatic intent of the writers behind their early texts might be. Consider the "message" behind the following text from a typical first grade basal reader:

> Ray loads the boat. He says, "I'll row."
> Neal says, "We'll both row."
> They leave, and Eve rides home alone.
> Neal and Ray see Eve ride. Neal waves. He and Ray row the boat home.
> (from *The Blue Book*, Headway Program, Open Court Publishing, 1979)

This is not a text with a clear or captivating communicative intent. The representation of conversation is thoroughly unconvincing, and totally redundant material is included. In fact, it is a "fake" text, in that its primary purpose is not actually to communicate anything the reader needs or wants to know, but to provide practice in reading by being easy to read. Nor is it atypical of basal readers.

Well, one might argue, so what? Children do need easy texts if they are to learn to read. Why should that purpose be puzzling to them? Of course, it is not puzzling to all children; many have successfully learned to read from texts just like this. I would argue, however, that these successful children have a previous understanding that texts are meant to communicate meaning and are thus able to be forgiving when confronted with uninteresting or meaningless texts. However, if the only forms of literacy children are exposed to consist of texts like this, and the accompanying worksheets, then they might well be excused for failing to understand that texts have authors behind them who are using literacy to try to express important meanings and have an impact on the world.

Many primary classrooms nowadays introduce literacy, not through reading, but through writing. Children are encouraged to write their own stories, using invented spelling, and then to read those stories aloud (Graves, 1978). Regularized versions of the child-written texts are used as the early books in reading lessons—texts that are read and discussed in the presence of their authors, so that the motivating communicative intent cannot be forgotten.

The success of such "writing before reading" methods for teaching literacy has been explained in a number of ways: It is easier to discover segmentation and the alphabetic principle from spelling than from word-reading (Read, 1986); motivation is higher (Bissex, 1980); and instruction by this method is more individualized. I would argue that the primary advantage such methods offer is they reduce the differences between oral and literate uses of language in the expression of communicative intents.

Children from homes in which parents have little education and low levels of literacy use are known to be at greater risk for failure at school, despite the fact that their oral language skills are perfectly adequate. For such children, a first confrontation with reading materials at school might be quite puzzling because they do not arrive at school already understanding that texts are meant to express meanings. As I have already argued, the earliest literacy experiences in traditional classrooms that rely on basal readers and worksheets may not clarify the potential of literacy to convey interesting messages. Children who come from literate households, on the other hand, arrive at school with considerable prior information about the potential of literacy to convey information, provide entertainment, and reflect their own important feelings (see, for example, Wolf & Heath, 1992, for case studies of two such highly literate children). Experiences of reading and discussing storybooks with adults, and of using books and newspapers as sources of information, may relate to success in the acquisition of literacy (Cochran-Smith, 1986; Goldfield & Snow, 1984; Teale, 1984) because they provide some children with a rich understanding that texts, like talk, can be used to do things in the world.

Another group of children at risk of failing at literacy are children who arrive at school speaking a language other than that used as the medium of instruction. If these children are taught to read in English, a language which they control minimally if at all, then they have no chance to discover the communicative potential of literacy, since what they are reading makes little sense to them. Children taught to read in a language they do not yet speak well show persistent academic difficulties, even if they are middle class and from educated families (Collier, 1987); these persistent problems may well relate to the obstacles these children face in understanding what reading is for and how it relates to real communication.

Conversation

Conversational rules constitute another domain in which children might be said to be precocious in their oral language accomplishments. Long before they can use language to express very complicated intents or meanings, infants engage in "proto-conversations" with adults in which they observe the rules of turn taking (Snow, 1977). Of course, adults help young children a lot in conversational exchanges—asking questions so that children have many opportunities to succeed in taking their turns, asking clarification questions or providing glosses for child utterances to ensure their content becomes part of the conversation, expanding on minimal child contributions to the conversation so their value is enhanced, following the child's lead in topic selection, and so on. This style of parent–child conversation, which is typical at least of middle-class American households, has been called "child-raising and self-lowering" (Ochs & Schieffelin, 1984); it is often referred to as "scaffolded conversation" to highlight how easy it makes the child's task of following conversational rules.

One advantage to the child of participating in conversation is that with the collaboration of the interlocutor, fairly complex messages can be conveyed. For example, stories of events that the child him- or herself would be unable to narrate clearly or unambiguously emerge as intelligible and complete because of adult questions and prompts and because adults fill in crucial information, ignore mistakes, and respond supportively.

Writing typically involves producing a message for a distant audience, usually without access to the sort of support that conversational partners provide. It is, then, not surprising that children's early attempts at writing connected discourse are relatively unsuccessful unless scaffolded by pictures or by access to reader responses. Many writing-based reading programs incorporate journals, which provide opportunities for children to write and receive relatively immediate response from adults (Peyton, 1986, 1988). Journals afford children one sort of transition between the situation of face-to-face conversation and the situation of writing for a distant audience. Other sorts of transitions are possible; when my son was six, he often initiated conversations in writing and greatly enjoyed participating in lengthy, face-to-face, but written exchanges (see Figure 12–1 for examples). These exchanges can be seen as a way of fracturing literacy into its components, accepting its print basis but rejecting its use for distanced communication.

An enormous advantage of face-to-face conversation is that speaker stance toward the message can be conveyed fairly easily and typically nonlin-

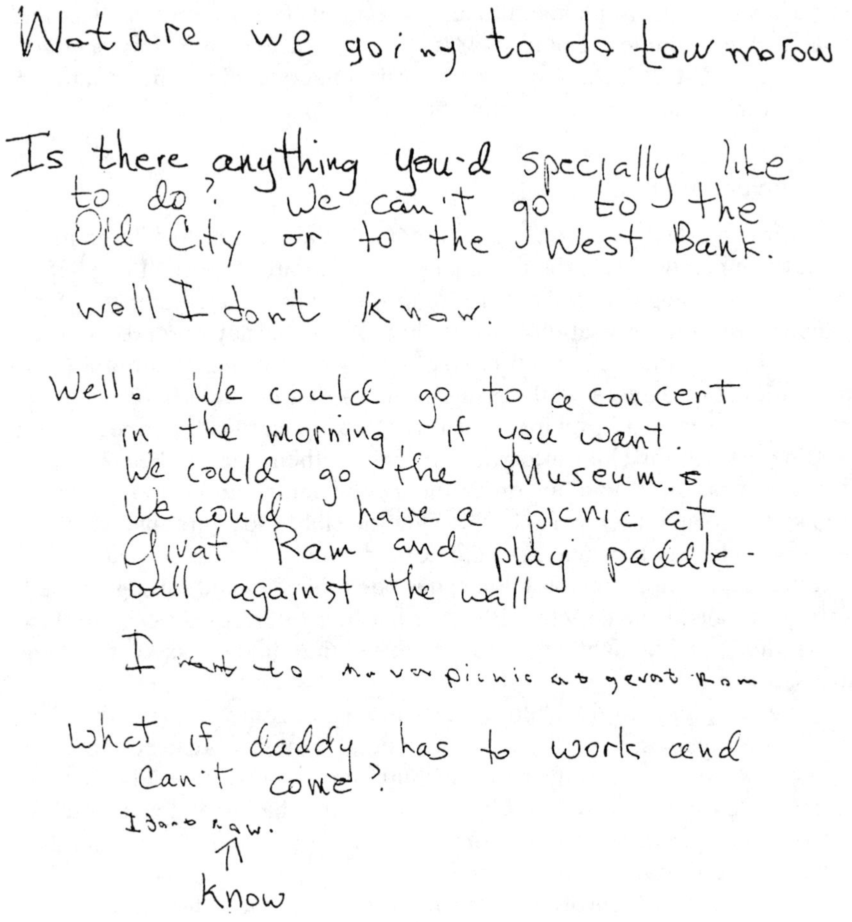

Wot are we going to do tow morow

Is there anything you'd specially like
to do? We can't go to the
Old City or to the West Bank.

well I don't know.

Well! We could go to a concert
in the morning, if you want.
We could go the Museum.s
We could have a picnic at
Givat Ram and play paddle-
ball against the wall

I want to no ver picnic at gevat Ram

What if daddy, has to work and
can't come?

I don't now.
          ↑
        know

FIGURE 12-1 Two examples of "written conversations" between a six-year-old and
his mother, demonstrating the boy's use of the literate mode to engage
in face-to-face conversation

anD its stil Boreeng
Is it boring because you
can't see or because the
music isn't very good? no its
Beecas i cant unDrstad
wat th man is saeing
The next piece they won't
talk — you just look at
the pictures. I stil wins
its Doreeng
andenywase i Dont
know wats
happeeng i the
picshr wen
i look at it

guistically or paralinguistically. Thus, the most affectively loaded utterances in a story can be produced with stress, or in a marked tone of voice, or with accompanying gestures. Such mechanisms are unavailable in writing, although unsophisticated writers often use graphic analogues like capitals, underlining, or exclamation points. More sophisticated writers substitute linguistic devices, such as unusual vocabulary items, metaphor, alliteration, or particular syntactic structures to highlight certain parts of their messages and make explicit their own stance toward the message. If readers are to understand the meaning of these devices when they encounter them in text, they must abandon the pragmatics of face-to-face conversation for the pragmatics of distanced communication.

Discourse

The pragmatics of connected discourse have to do with the relations across utterances—making clear how propositions are tied together. Cross-utterance connections can be quite complex. How should one best present the various events that constitute the background to a narrative? Or the various steps in an argument or an explanation? Consider the following example of a possible conversation:

A: John doesn't seem to have any love interest recently.
B: He's been visiting San Francisco quite a lot.

Does B's response constitute an agreement with A's claim through a suggestion that John has been compensating for celibacy by engaging in sight-seeing, or a counterclaim that he has a nonlocal love interest? If this were an oral exchange, tone of voice and intonation might disambiguate the intent. And if for some reason it didn't, then A could always query B, "You mean he's seeing someone there?" Or if A misinterpreted B's response, there would still be a chance for conversational repair:

A: Who is he seeing in San Francisco?
B: He's not seeing *anyone* there. He goes and rides cable cars to console himself.

Needless to say, such query and repair mechanisms are unavailable in distanced and literate communication. B would need to be much more explicit in the second sentence:

A tells me John isn't seeing anyone these days. Instead, he's been visiting San Francisco quite a lot. He goes there to ride cable cars to combat his loneliness.

or

A tells me John isn't seeing anyone these days. But he has been visiting San Francisco quite a lot. I wonder if he doesn't have a friend there none of us knows about.

Satisfying the pragmatic demands of distanced communication requires predicting what sorts of information the distant audience will need to know, and what sorts of misinterpretations they might be inclined to make. Thus, effective distanced communication requires planning and prediction, since the interlocutor is not available to help one fine tune one's message. But young children are used to communicating with listeners who are not distant—people in the same room, and people with whom they share a considerable amount of background knowledge. They are also used to being able to enter a conversation in the middle, without themselves linguistically providing all the background information that would help situate their remarks. The pragmatics of communicating with familiar, physically present interlocutors who already know a good deal about what you want to tell them versus that with unfamiliar, physically distant listeners who may or may not share background knowledge with you are quite different. It is not surprising if children fall back on the pragmatics of the more frequently encountered situation when in fact a novel pragmatics is needed. Examples of attempts to accommodate to the demands of distanced communication, also from my son but at ages 9 and 11, are presented in Figures 12–2 and 12–3. Neither is completely incomprehensible, but both are situated in personal or historical contexts in ways that compromise full accessibility for the relative stranger. The first relates an incident with his grandparents (Lyle is his grandmother) and shows some tension in the choice of tenses between presenting generic aspects of their relationship and a specific event. The second is a comment on an event of some currency at the time of writing, but it shows little awareness of the likelihood that it might be read in a historical context when this particular conflict between the United States and Libya is no longer a major issue.

An additional source of evidence that young children have problems with the pragmatics of distanced communication, rather than with the challenge of literacy per se, comes from work on referential communication tasks, in which children consistently have trouble understanding the need to predict the likelihood of miscommunication. Having come up with a description for one target (e.g., a picture of a nonsense object) that seems appropriate, children are less likely than adults to check whether it could also apply to another possible target, or whether its interpretation relies on knowledge that the interlocutor cannot obtain. Thus their messages are typically idiosyncratic and insufficiently informative (Glucksberg & Krauss, 1967; Sonnenschein & Whitehurst, 1984). Furthermore, somewhat older children who understand that they must adjust their messages to the needs of an absent audience still do not always succeed in making the most appropriate adjustments (De Temple, Wu, & Snow, 1991). For example, they produce longer descriptions for a distant uninformed audience, but not necessarily clearer or more interpretable descriptions.

Figures 12–2 and 12–3 give examples of failure by a young writer to accommodate to the pragmatics of distanced communication. But failure in writing is not the only issue—young children need to **comprehend** the pragmatics of distancing as well. Much of what structures written text is, in fact,

United States and Libya

I think that it was actualy our and Western Europes fault because before like 50 years ago they wanted to own it and they didn't much care for the Arabs so they told the Jewish (who needed a place to go) to go and take some of that land. They also said that nobody lived there but actually the Arabs lived there. The jewish moved in and had a war with the Arabs. The jewish won, got more land, and the Arabs started terrorist attacks against the Jewish and the Americans. They were against the Americans because the Americans supported Isreal in the wars. Now they have terrorist attacks against us and after what just happened there will be more terrorists attacks.

by Nathaniel Baumdrow

FIGURE 12-2   An essay written by an eleven-year-old for a social studies current events assignment

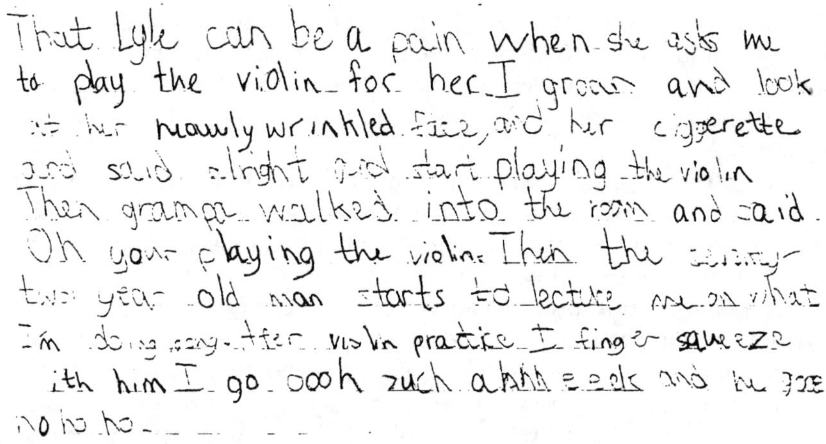

That Lyle can be a pain when she asks me
to play the violin for her I groan and look
at her mealy wrinkled face, and her cigerette
and said alright and start playing the violin
Then grampa walked into the room and said.
Oh your playing the violin. Then the seventy-
two year old man starts to lecture me on what
I'm doing wrong. After violin practice I finger squeeze
with him I go oooh zuch ahhh eeek and he goe
ho ho ho - - - - -

FIGURE 12–3 An essay written by a nine-year-old boy about a visit to his grandparents

accommodation to the peculiar pragmatics of distanced communication between relatively unfamiliar interlocutors. It is not surprising if young children who have not practiced and do not control those pragmatics in their own production are somewhat baffled when they encounter them in their reading.

CONVERSATION VERSUS CONNECTED DISCOURSE AND LITERACY

I have argued that the pragmatics of oral language use cannot be transferred easily to literacy, and that the problems children encounter in acquiring literacy may be traceable to their presumption that oral language pragmatics apply in literate contexts. Data supporting this claim come from two sources: differential relationships between skill in oral language tasks and in literacy, and data suggesting that experiences that promote skill with distanced communication also promote literacy outcomes.

Conversations versus Definitions

In a study of various language skills and their relation to literacy, carried out with children at the United Nations International School (UNIS), we attempted to assess performance on language tasks that differed in their pragmatic demands. The children in the study were second through fifth graders, and they were all to some extent bilingual, either because their home language was not English (the medium of instruction at UNIS) or because at UNIS they had studied French as a foreign language. Thus, we could test not just the associations across language tasks in these children, but also the associations within the same task across performance in two languages.

An intriguing finding emerged from this study differentiating two types of language tasks: carrying on conversations and giving definitions. I will first summarize the facts about the administration of and results from each task, then contrast them explicitly.

The conversation task (Schley & Snow, 1992) required the child to interview the adult, as if for a television talk show. Children were instructed to act like talk-show hosts, and to ask questions about any topic they wanted, including books, movies, work, recreation, vacations, trips, and so on. They were told to keep the conversation going for four minutes; the adults responded appropriately but not effusively to child questions and topic initiations, so as to make the task somewhat challenging. Indicators of performance on this task differentiated the children into three groups:

1. The very competent performers initiated topics with open-ended questions and tended to continue a topic by expanding on the adult's response, rather than initiating new topics with every exchange. These children also had few silences or filled pauses in their talk.
2. The middle group asked many more yes–no or short-answer questions of the adult and were more likely to ask a whole list of unrelated questions than to ask follow-up questions. They were as fluent as the first group.
3. The group identified as very poor at the interview task failed to ask open-ended or follow-up questions and also displayed high levels of dysfluency, with many silent and filled pauses in their speech.

Interestingly, although there was some tendency for the fifth graders to be better than the second graders, there was not a very strong or consistent set of age differences on this task; individual differences in performance were considerably larger than age effects. Although exposure to English in the home related to performance on the conversation task in English, performance was not necessarily worse in a second than a first language; in fact, on a number of measures children performed better in French (which they had studied as a foreign language) than in English, perhaps because they could draw upon the dialogues they studied and practiced in French class. Most striking was how challenging this task was for children—in fact, it is a task that many adults have not fully mastered, perhaps because doing it well is simply quite difficult. Despite the large component of intelligent strategizing which is prerequisite to success on this task, performance does not correlate with any indicator of school achievement and shows no relationship to literacy.

TABLE 12-2 Comparison of Conversation and Definitions Tasks

	CONVERSATION	DEFINITIONS
DEVELOPS BETWEEN 7-12 YEARS	Some development, large individual differences	Considerable development during school years
TASK DIFFICULTY	High; persistent problems in adulthood	Minimal; simple form with little variation
L1-L2 CORRELATIONS	Moderate	Absent unless schooled in both languages
SES DIFFERENCES	Untested	Present in kindergarten-aged children
MEASURABLE HOME LANGUAGE INFLUENCE?	Performance better in home language	Performance not better in language used at home
MEASURABLE SCHOOL LANGUAGE INFLUENCE?	Small effect of use of language in school, especially if taught	Performance directly correlated with school use of language
CORRELATED TO LITERACY?	No correlation	Highly correlated

A second task carried out with the UNIS children involved giving definitions of simple words—nail, umbrella, bicycle, and so on. Since the words were common and well known, this was not in any sense a vocabulary test; rather, children's responses were scored to reflect the degree to which they conformed to the standards of "good," formal, Aristotelian definitions (Snow, 1990). Performance on the definitions task showed robust age effects, with the second graders producing approximately 50 percent formal definitions and the fifth graders almost 90 percent. The best predictor of performance on definitions in English was history of schooling in English; surprisingly, exposure to English in the home was not related to performance on this task, and there were no correlations between how well the children performed the task in French and in English. Most striking, though, were the robust correlations between performance on the definitions task and literacy scores (Snow, Cancino, Gonzalez, & Shriberg, 1989).

Table 12-2 presents a brief and oversimplified contrast between the definitions task and the conversation task on a number of salient dimensions. The conversation task is more challenging, less influenced by age or experience in school, and uncorrelated with literacy. The definitions task is obviously simpler, more susceptible to an orderly influence of age and school experiences, affected by social class (Dickinson & Snow, 1987), and strongly correlated to literacy. Why these differences?

I would argue that definitions relate to literacy at least in part because "solving" the definitions task requires analyzing the peculiar pragmatic demands of the definition genre (Snow, Cancino, De Temple, & Schley, 1991).

The genre is characterized not just by a particular syntactic structure but also by the presumption of distanced communication and the need for explicit provision of what might in fact be shared information. Thus, pointing to the experimenter's watch is an inadequate response to the question "What is a watch?" under the rules of giving definitions; saying "an apparatus worn on the wrist and used to tell time" is required even when an ostensive definition might be interpersonally perfectly appropriate and communicatively more effective. Children who have figured out the pragmatics of definitions are probably sensitive to the somewhat opaque pragmatics of literacy forms as well, practiced in the explicit provision of information, and skilled in avoiding the presumption of shared background knowledge. The conversation task is challenging and no doubt related to success in some important domains of human competence, but solving it does not require any particular skill in the pragmatics of distanced communication.

Predictors of Literacy in Oral Language

If doing well in the definitions task is a proxy for understanding the pragmatics of distanced discourse because control over the pragmatics of distanced communication underlie both, then in what contexts do children acquire these pragmatic skills? What social–interactive experiences help children to acquire the relevant insights and experience? David Dickinson, Patton Tabors, and I are attempting to answer this question through the Home-School Study of Language and Literacy Development; this is a longitudinal study of low-income childen, that is, those who are at some risk of failing to achieve satisfactory literacy outcomes (Snow, 1991b; Snow & Dickinson, 1991). By assessing the nature of the language interactions these children have access to at home and in their preschools, we hope to be able to identify the contexts within which they acquire skills with distanced, explicit communication.

One place we are starting is by assessing the children's exposure to connected discourse. So, for example, we have found that the frequency of narratives in the families' dinner table conversations when the children are three or four relates to their comprehension of stories at age five, and that the amount of topic-expanding, nonimmediate talk their mothers engage in while reading a book to the children at three and four predicts the children's preliteracy skills (De Temple & Beals, 1991; Dickinson & Tabors, 1991). In preschools as well, opportunities for exposure to connected discourse, whether in adult-dominated contexts like book reading and circle time or in peer interactions, relate to language and literacy outcomes for these high-risk children (Dickinson & Smith, 1991; see also Dickinson, Chapter 13).

The Home-School Study will continue to follow children through grade 4—the point at which the reading skills of poor children are often revealed as inadequate to the demands of school literacy. We expect the relationship between distanced oral language skills and literacy outcomes to strengthen as children get older, because the effectiveness of projecting the pragmatics of oral face-to-face communication onto literacy declines as literacy tasks become more challenging.

CONCLUSION

It has been my goal in this chapter to demonstrate how the pragmatics of face-to-face communication fail when extrapolated oversimplistically to the sort of distanced communication that is typical of literacy. Although the most obvious difference between oral and literate uses of language might seem to relate to the use of print for literacy, I have argued that print is much less a problem than pragmatics. The pragmatics of spoken language used for face-to-face communication are very complex, and children who master them certainly possess sufficient cognitive and linguistic sophistication to deal with distanced pragmatics as well. But they must be given the opportunity to learn how distanced, literate communication differs from face-to-face, oral communication. If we do not provide those opportunities, then we should not be surprised if children have problems learning to read.

NOTE

The generous support of the Ford Foundation and the Spencer Foundation to the Home-School Study of Language and Literacy Development, in the context of which many of the ideas presented in this paper were developed, is gratefully acknowledged. I am also grateful to David Dickinson and Patton Tabors, collaborators on the Home-School Study.

REFERENCES

Adams, M. J. (1990). *Beginning to read: Thinking and learning about print.* Cambridge, MA: MIT Press.

Austin, J. L. (1962). *How to do things with words.* Cambridge, MA: Harvard University Press.

Bissex, G. (1980). *Gnys at wrk.* Cambridge, MA: Harvard University Press.

Bradley, L., & Bryant, P. (1985). *Rhyme and reason in reading and spelling.* Ann Arbor, MI: University of Michigan Press.

Brown, P., & Levinson, S. (1978). Universals in language usage: Politeness phenomena. In E. Goody (Ed.), *Questions and politeness: Strategies in social interaction* (pp. 56–289). New York: Cambridge University Press.

Cochran-Smith, M. (1986). Reading to children: A model for understanding texts. In B. Schieffelin & P. Gilmore (Eds.), *The acquisition of literacy: Ethnographic perspectives* (pp. 35–54). Norwood, NJ: Ablex.

Collier, V. (1987). Age and rate of acquisition of second language for academic purposes. *TESOL Quarterly 21*, 617–641.

De Temple, J., & Beals, D. (1991). Family talk: Sources of support for the development of decontextualized language skills. *Journal of Research in Childhood Education, 6*, 11–19.

De Temple, J., Wu, H F., & Snow, C. E. (1991). Papa Pig just left for Pigtown: Children's oral and written picture descriptions under varying instructions. *Discourse Processes, 14*, 469–495.

Dickinson, D. K., & Smith, M. (1991). Preschool talk: Patterns of teacher–child interaction in early childhood classrooms. *Journal of Research in Childhood Education, 6*, 20–29.

Dickinson, D. K., & Snow, C. E. (1987). Interrelationships among prereading and oral language skills in kindergartners from two social classes. *Research on Childhood Education Quarterly, 2*, 1–25.

Dickinson, D. K., & Tabors, P. O. (1991). Early literacy: Linkages between home, school, and literacy achievement at age five. *Journal of Research in Childhood Education, 6*, 30–46.

Dore, J. (1974). A pragmatic description for early languge development. *Journal of Psycholinguistic Research, 4*, 343–350.

Dore, J. (1975). Holophrases, speech acts and language universals. *Journal of Child Language, 2*, 21–40.

Ehri, L. C. (1984). How orthography alters spoken language competencies in children learning to read and spell. In J. Downing & R. Valtin (Eds.), *Language awareness and learning to read* (pp. 119–148). New York: Springer-Verlag.

Glucksberg, S., & Krauss, R. (1967). What do people say after they have learned how to talk? *Merrill-Palmer Quarterly, 13*, 309–316.

Goldfield, B. A., & Snow, C. E. (1984). Reading books with children: The mechanics of parental influence on children's reading achievement. In J. Flood (Ed.), *Promoting reading comprehension* (pp. 204–215). Newark, DE: International Reading Association.

Graves, D. H. (1978). *Balance the basics: Let them write.* New York: Ford Foundation.

Hayes, D., & Ahrens, M. (1988). Vocabulary simplification for children. *Journal of Child Language, 15*, 457–472.

Helfgott, J. (1976). Phoneme segmentation and blending skills of kindergarten children: Implications for beginning reading acquistion. *Contemporary Education Psychology, 1*, 157–169.

Liberman, I. Y., Shankweiler, D., Liberman, A. M., Fowler, C., & Fischer, F. W. (1977). Phonetic segmentation and recording in the beginning reader. In A. S. Reber & D. L. Scarborough (Eds.), *Toward a psychology of reading* (pp. 207–226). Hillsdale, NJ: Lawrence Erlbaum.

Mann, V. A. (1991). Language problems: A key to early reading problems. In B. Y. L. Wong (Ed.), *Learning about learning disabilites* (pp. 129–162). New York: Academic Press.

Ninio, A., & Snow, C. E. (1988). Language acquisition through language use: The functional sources of children's early utterances. In Y. Levy, I. Schlesinger, & M. Braine (Eds.), *Categories and processes in language acquisition* (pp. 11–30). Hillsdale, NJ: Lawrence Erlbaum.

Ochs, E., & Schieffelin, B. B. (1984). Language acquisition and socialization: Three developmental stories and their implications. In R. A. Shweder & R. A. Levine (Eds.), *Culture theory: Essays on mind, self, and emotion* (pp. 276–320). New York: Cambridge University Press.

Peyton, J. K. (1986). Literacy through written interaction. *Passage, 2*(1), 24–29.

Peyton, J. K. (1988). *The effect of teacher strategies on students' interactive writing: The case of dialogue journals.* UCLA: Center for Language Education and Research.

Read, C. (1975). *Children's categorization of speech sounds in English.* NCTE (Research Rep. No. 17). Urbana, IL: National Council of Teachers of English.

Read, C. (1986). *Children's creative spelling.* London: Routledge and Kegan Paul.

Ryan, E. B., & Ledger, G. W. (1984). Learning to attend to sentence structure: Links between metalinguistic development and reading. In J. Downing & R. Valtin (Eds.), *Language awareness and learning to read* (pp. 149–172). New York: Springer-Verlag.

Searle, J. (1969). *Speech acts: An essay in the philosophy of language.* New York: Cambridge University Press.

Schley, S., & Snow, C. E. (1992). The conversational skills of school-aged children. *Social Development, 1,* 18–35.

Snow, C. E. (1977). Development of conversation between mothers and babies. *Journal of Child Language, 4,* 1–22.

Snow, C. E. (1990). The development of definitional skill. *Journal of Child Language, 17,* 697–710.

Snow, C. E. (1991a). Language proficiency: Towards a definition. In H. Dechert & G. Appel (Eds.), *A case for psycholinguistic cases* (pp. 63–89). Hilversum, Netherlands: John Benjamins.

Snow, C. E. (1991b). The theoretical basis for relationships between language and literacy development. *Journal of Research in Childhood Education, 6,* 5–10.

Snow, C. E., Cancino, H., De Temple, J., & Schley, S. (1991). Giving formal definitions: A linguistic or metalinguistic skill? In E. Bialystok (Ed.), *Language processing and language awareness by bilingual children* (pp. 90–112). New York: Cambridge University Press.

Snow, C., Cancino, H., Gonzalez, P., & Shriberg, E. (1989). Giving formal definitions: An oral language correlate of school literacy. In D. Bloome (Ed.), *Classrooms and literacy* (pp. 233–249). Norwood, NJ: Ablex.

Snow, C. E., & Dickinson, D. K. (1991). Skills that aren't basic in a new conception of literacy. In A. Purves & T. Jennings (Eds.), *Literate systems and individual lives: Perspectives on literacy and schooling* (pp. 179–191). Albany, NY: SUNY Press.

Snow, C. E., & Tabors, P. O. (in press). Language skills that relate to literacy development. In B. Spodek & O. Saracho (Eds.), *Yearbook in early childhood education* (Vol. 4, B). New York: Teachers College Press.

Sonnenschein, S., & Whitehurst, G. (1984). Developing referential communication: A hierarchy of skills. *Child Development, 55,* 1936–1945.

Teale, W. H. (1984). Reading to young children: Its significance for literacy development. In H. Goelman, A. Oberg, & F. Smith (Eds.), *Awakening to literacy* (pp. 110–122). Exeter, NH: Heinemann Educational Books.

Treiman, R., & Baron, J. (1981). Segmental analysis ability: Development and relation to reading ability. In G. E. MacKinnon and T. G. Walker (Eds.), *Reading research: Advances in theory and practice* (Vol. 3, pp. 159–198). New York: Academic Press.

Vellutino, F. R., & Scallon, D. (1987). Phonological coding, phonological awareness, and reading ability: Evidence from longitudinal and experimental study. *Merrill-Palmer Quarterly, 33,* 321–363.

Wolf, S. A., & Heath, S. B. (1992). *The braid of literature: Children's worlds of reading.* Cambridge, MA: Harvard University Press.

chapter 13

FEATURES OF EARLY CHILDHOOD CLASSROOM ENVIRONMENTS THAT SUPPORT DEVELOPMENT OF LANGUAGE AND LITERACY

David K. Dickinson

The goal of "fostering language development" carries diverse meanings for different teachers—meanings that depend on the long-term goals they hold for children. For some severely challenged children, establishing language as a medium for meaningful communication is the ultimate objective. For others, it is hoped that oral language skills will provide a foundation for literacy. It is necessary to bear in mind these long-term language-related objectives when planning classroom language programs, because oral language is used for many purposes and some of them are more likely to foster acquisition of literacy-related skills than are others. My research has been done in classrooms serving children who are developing language normally in which the teachers are concerned with fostering academic skills; therefore my discussion focuses on ways in which classrooms can support literacy-related aspects of language skill.

As Snow (Chapter 12) explains in more detail, analyses of varying kinds of written language have found that certain important uses (e.g., communicating novel information, arguing a point of view) tend to result in linguistic forms and interactional strategies that are quite different from those used in the context of informal conversations between friends (see also Chafe, 1985; Dickinson, 1987). Such types of written language place a premium on communicating information explicitly (i.e., using words and syntax rather than intonation, gesture, and allusion to shared knowledge) and rely on extended discourse to communicate meaning. Although these differences are clearest when extremely divergent kinds of oral and written language are compared (e.g., written essay vs. informal conversation), they also can be used to distinguish among ways of using language within a given modality. For example, if we consider only oral language, some topics (e.g., communication of complex novel information) and situations (e.g., minimal shared background knowledge, inability to use gestures) create conditions that lead to the use of more explicit and elaborative oral language forms.

When people engage in conversations, they develop many subtle techniques for entertaining, for narrating experiences, and for convincing others of positions they hold. Unfortunately, the strategies honed through interpersonal conversations are not necessarily the same as those required for engaging in the type of literacy activity valued and assessed in schools in Western technological societies. In order to be successful at literacy tasks in this context, children need access to strategies that enable them to communicate novel information explicitly. Therefore, it is not surprising that children who are skilled conversationalists are not necessarily skilled readers and writers (Snow, Cancino, Gonzalez, & Shriberg, 1989; Torrance & Olson, 1985). Instead, skill using oral language in ways consistent with the manner required for discursive written language is what counts when children approach literacy tasks. The implication of this finding is clear: Teachers who are interested in building oral language supports for literacy need to make special efforts to create activities that support the kinds of oral language skills likely to foster long-term literacy development.

A FRAMEWORK FOR EXAMINING CLASSROOM INTERACTIONAL SETTINGS

Language is produced in social settings to achieve certain ends. If teachers wish to encourage children to practice using literacy-related oral language, they need to consider three intertwined aspects of the interactional setting: (1) enduring aspects of the **relationship** between the speaker and hearer, including such features as status difference and social distance; (2) the general type of **classroom activity** (e.g., meeting time, snack time); and (3) the immediate short-term **agendas** of the interactants. These variables affect who does the talking, who controls the topic, and the general content of the talk (e.g., explanations, instructions). In addition to these environmental issues, teachers need to take into account a fourth variable, the **developmental level** of their children.

In the first portion of this chapter, I present data showing how these features of classrooms tend to shape the nature of language used in early childhood programs. Next, I report data showing the impact of certain types of classroom discourse on long-term development of vocabulary and language comprehension. Finally, I close with some practical suggestions for classroom teachers.

Speaker–Hearer Relationship

One important way of categorizing speaker–hearer relationships in preschools is in terms of whether the child's conversational partner is a peer or an adult. For the past four years a team of researchers at Clark and Harvard Universities directed by Catherine Snow and myself has been following the language and literacy development of a group of low-income children (i.e., those eligible for Head Start). One facet of this project has included audio-taping three- and four-year-old children's conversations during the morning in preschool classrooms. Half of our children are in Head Start classrooms and the remainder are in other classrooms that serve some low-income children. We have coded children's conversations for the general content of the talk, for whether the child is speaking with an adult or with another child, and for the general kind of activity (e.g., free time, group time). Each interaction is timed, allowing us to determine in seconds the amount of time children engaged in varied types of interactions during the morning.

Categories used to code the interactions included the following:

Pretending: fantasy-oriented talk

Nonpresent talk: talk about the past (e.g., personal narratives) or talk about the future (e.g., planning)

Conceptual focus: talk with requirements for understanding that include world knowledge (e.g., scientific, historical, current events) and talk about language (e.g., word meanings)

Book reading: reading and talking about books

Didactic talk: talk providing instructions and procedural information and explanations regarding appropriate behavior ("don't hit him because it will hurt")

Skill routines: language routines familiar to all participants, including reciting numbers and letters and singing

Print skills: talk about print, decoding, rhyming, spelling, and child dictations

Control talk: talk designed to manage behavior

Engaged talk: general conversation not captured by other categories (e.g., personal preferences, talk about the backpack worn by the child)

Nonlanguage: all interactions during which bursts of talk around a single topic last less than 5 seconds; gross motor activity unaccompanied by talk

As shown in Table 13–1, the identity of the interactant has a major impact on the content of the talk. Our coding of all of our target child's interactions throughout a morning indicates that when children are with other children, they are quite likely to engage in pretend talk. When they are with adults their conversations take a much more instructional focus. When interacting with three-year-olds, teachers spend more time socializing behavior

TABLE 13–1 Correlations between Percentage of Time Recorded Interacting with Different Partners and Percentage of Time Observed Engaging in Different Types of Talk at Two Ages

Talk Types	AGE THREE (n = 25)		
	Alone	With Child	With Adult
Pretending		.80[3]	−.31
Didactic	−.56[b]		.58[b]
Control	−.35		.41[a]
Engaged talk	−.43[a]		.36
Skill routines	−.38[a]	−.33	.49[b]
Nonlanguage	.93[d]		−.82[d]

Talk Types	AGE FOUR (n = 36)		
	Alone	With Child	With Adult
Print skills	−.36[a]		.56[c]
Pretending	−.53[b]	.83[d]	

[a]p<.05
[b]p<.01
[c]p<.001
[d]p<.0001

("didactic" and "control") and helping children practice familiar routines; when teachers interacted with four-year-olds, they tended to spend time on print-related knowledge. These patterns strongly indicate that when children talk with adults, the adults tend to select the topic, determine the direction of the conversation, and produce the most talk. When children are with other children, the talk quickly enters the fantasy realm in which children mutually determine and develop topics (see Dickinson & Smith, 1991, for additional details).

We have not charted other ways in which aspects of speaker–hearer identities influence interaction in classrooms, but I have no doubt that many other features of identities can influence interactions. For example, children are almost certain to engage in different kinds of pretending with different partners and they may differ in how they interact with various adults who may spend time in the room.

Classroom Activity

A second factor with a major impact on the nature of classroom language is the activity and the roles that teachers assume during them. Activity settings are critical to consider because they determine who and how many interactants are involved, the roles they assume, and activity-specific expectations governing behavior (e.g., what is discussed, how turns are allocated, etc.). Classroom

TABLE 13–2 Correlations between Percentages of Time Recorded Engaging in Different Types of Talk and Percentage of Time Spent in Different Types of Activities at Two Ages

	AGE THREE (n = 25)	
Talk Types	Free Play	Full Group
Skill routines		.80[d]
Conceptual focus		−.37[a]
Pretend	.43[a]	

	AGE FOUR (n = 37)	
Talk Types	Free Play	Full Group
Print skills	−.46[b]	.49[b]
Skill routines	−.33[a]	.39[b]
Engaged talk	.55[c]	

[a]p<.05
[b]p<.01
[c]p<.001
[d]p<.0001

activity also is interesting because it is a central way in which teachers conceptualize their day.

Activity type. One broad way of classifying classroom activities is in terms of whether children are in a free play type of setting or in a more structured group meeting. "Free play" does not describe the kind of activity a child actually engages in during a given time, but it is the type of designation teachers use for time blocks. While "full group" time is more standardized in early childhood settings—often including talk about the calendar, some talk about coming activities, and reading one or more books—the content of full group times also varies greatly from one teacher to the next.

The audiotapes made in preschool classrooms collected as part of our ongoing study of language and literacy development provide evidence of the impact of classroom activity type on children's language. As shown in Table 13–2, at both ages children are more likely to be engaged in skill-related talk if they spend more time in full group settings. Children in classrooms with more time set for free play are more likely to engage in pretending when they are three and more likely to engage in general conversations when they are four. One feature of these results worthy of special note is the fact that although there are general linkages between the content of children's conversations and classroom activity, the amount of time allocated to free play is only loosely related to the amount of time children engage in pretending. Given that free play is a time when children can play with others and given the strong association between time spent with children and amount of pre-

TABLE 13–3 Proportion of Utterances Reflecting Conversation about Nonpresent Topics When Teachers Working with the Same Group of Four-Year-Olds Were Circulating or Stationary during Choice Time and during Lunch Time

TEACHER	STATIONARY	CIRCULATING	LUNCH TIME
Connie	(n = 172)	(n = 101)	(n = 142)
	.42	.14	.14
Terri	(n = 122)	(n = 226)	(n = 80)
	.48	.29	.22
Petra	(n = 118)	(n = 118)	(n = 143)
	.51	.26	.30

tending, one might anticipate a stronger association between time spent in free play and pretending. The relatively weak link between pretending and amount of free play time points to the fact that time blocks only provide opportunities for given types of interactions to occur. To ensure that the types of activities that are desirable (e.g., pretending) actually occur, teachers need to attend to the organization of the environment and they need to encourage valued behaviors.

Teacher role within an activity. Even during a given type of activity, teacher–child interaction is affected by the role that the teacher assumes within the activity. For example, during periods when children are free to engage in activities around the room, teachers may circulate from one area to another, or they may remain stationary in one location for a time. Built into these two patterns are distinct assumptions about the role of the teacher. The "floater" typically keeps children on task and intervenes to settle problems or to encourage continued engagement, while the stationary teacher may introduce an activity, keep children focused, and engage in conversations.

Evidence of the effect of these role designations on the kind of talk that occurs between teachers and children comes from a study in which three teachers, who worked with the same group of children, were audiotaped in their classroom on three different days. The tapes were transcribed and coded for the conversational topic of each utterance (see Dickinson, 1991, for a more complete description). Because of its likely long-term significance for literacy development, conversations were coded for talk that moved beyond the immediate context. Such "nonpresent" talk included analytical conversations (information about the world, talk about language) as well as talk about the future and the past. As shown in Table 13–3, teachers were two to three times more likely to engage in nonpresent talk with children when they stayed in one location than when they were circulating around the room.

Qualitative analyses indicated that these differences reflected different agendas: "floaters" kept the children engaged in the activities available in the room; stationary adults were available as conversational partners.

Teacher Agenda

In addition to structural and organizational factors that influence teacher–child talk, teachers may vary in terms of personal interactional styles. Personal styles have cultural roots (Michaels, 1991; Minami & McCabe, 1991), they may reflect pedagogical orientations derived from one's training, and they may reflect idiosyncratic personality differences. These factors have not been well investigated in classroom settings, but their influence was clearly shown in the previously discussed study of teacher–child interaction in preschool (Dickinson, 1991).

In that study, I examined teacher–child interaction during lunch times as well as during free times. Studies of meals at home have found them to be settings conducive to relaxed, extended talk, often rich with narratives and explanations (De Temple & Beals, 1991; Heath, 1986). To determine whether this is also true in classrooms, I audiotaped lunch time conversations between children and the three teachers who worked with them. Analysis of the transcripts of these tapes indicated, in general, even lower levels of extended nonpresent talk than was found during times when teachers were circulating around the room (see Table 13–3.) This finding further indicates the impact of activity type on interactions in classrooms. But the finding of immediate relevance was the fact that despite the generally low levels of nonpresent talk, there were interesting indications of differences associated with individual teachers' lunch time values.

One teacher, Terri, engaged in the least overall amount of talk and was concerned primarily with nutrition and table manners. Of the seven interactions that she initiated that lasted four or more speaking turns, two had to do with eating salad, four dealt with manners (e.g., how to ask for items on the table, to whom they should and should not talk during lunch), and one dealt with the upcoming potluck dinner. Children initiated only three topics, all of which involved requests for food or for permission to leave the table. In contrast, at the table where Petra was in charge, no interactions dealt strictly with manners, four dealt with management-related matters (e.g., completing the meal, eating salad), and six initiated nonpresent topics (e.g., weekend plans, discussion about the morning, query about why a child was being mean). The children also initiated a number of nonpresent topics. Furthermore, across the three lunch times that were recorded, children at Petra's table talked more than twice as much as those at Terri's table (158 vs. 62 utterances). Thus, working under the same functional constraints (i.e., same roles, same task to accomplish), these two teachers created vastly different interactional environments; one encouraged free-flowing and wide-ranging talk, while the other created an environment that was not conducive to such talk.

Developmental Level

The variables dealt with thus far all focus on the environment, but preschool teachers also are acutely aware of having to consider the needs of individual children. Nonetheless, in discussions about typical preschoolers, the "preschool years" (i.e., ages three and four) often are lumped together as if this is a relatively undifferentiated phase of development. However, these years span major growth in children's linguistic resources, including a flowering of pretending and much more ability to talk about past and future events (see Dickinson & McCabe, 1991, for a review). Data that we present later suggest that the kinds of activities that most support children's emerging language and literacy skills may well vary by age, with child–child interactions being most important for younger children and adult–child interactions playing a larger role for older children.

Other changes related to development that appear during these years occur as a result of shifting adult expectations that are driven by societally determined timetables. Teachers know that, in general, four-year-olds will enter kindergarten the following year and that literacy and numeracy play a major role in determining children's success. As a result, as we previously reported (see Table 13–2), teachers' priorities shift from primary concern with helping children learn to interact in organized group settings when they are three, to growing attention to skills related to the academic demands when they are four. These changes, reflected in changing patterns of correlation at the two ages (i.e., between activity type, time spent with adults, and topic content) clearly indicate that adults begin to focus increasingly on prereading skills as children get closer to entering kindergarten.

EFFECTS OF CLASSROOMS ON LANGUAGE AND EARLY LITERACY

We have argued that certain kinds of language skills are theoretically linked to later literacy development and that opportunities to practice those skills in early childhood classrooms are likely to be beneficial to children's long-term literacy development. Although these claims are based on good theory, it is reassuring to be able to report that we now have some empirical support for these claims.

When the children in the Home-School Study were five, we began giving them a battery of tests of language and literacy skills. Tests of early literacy skill come from the Early Childhood Diagnostic Inventory and include tests of ability to read environmental print (i.e., print seen on signs or labels), letter-naming ability, phonemic awareness, story and print concepts, and writing ability. Tests of receptive oral language skill include a test of vocabulary knowledge (Peabody Picture Vocabulary Test), and a test of story comprehension that involved asking children questions about a children's book, *The Snowy Day* by Ezra Jack Keats, as it was read to them by an experimenter. Productive language tasks included telling a story about a series of three pictures of teddy bears, describing a picture of a circus, and defining familiar words. Productive oral language tasks were scored for length and quality of response.[1] In the following discussion we report some of the results linking preschool experiences to kindergarten measures of language and literacy development using the proposed framework for examining language in preschoc: classrooms as an organizing framework (see Dickinson & ?.bors, 1991, for more detailed results).

Speaker–Hearer Relationship and Activity Type

In our analytic scheme the identity of the interactants and the nature of the activity can be distinguished, but in classrooms they are inextricably intertwined. Nonetheless, we did find one correlation between the identity of speakers and our outcome variables. For three-year-olds the percentage of time that we recorded children interacting with other children was strongly related to kindergarten scores on our vocabulary test ($r = .68$, $p < .001$), print skill ($r = .42$, $p < .05$), and story understanding ($r = .47$, $p < .01$). This powerful effect is largely explained by the fact that children usually engaged in pretend activities with other children and that the amount of time spent pretending was also strongly linked to our measures of vocabulary ($r = .59$, $p < .01$), print skill ($r = .54$, $p < .01$), and story understanding ($r = .46$, $p < .05$), and to the ability to define words (a measure of children's ability to talk about language) ($r = .43$, $p < .05$).

For four-year-olds the links between outcomes and classroom experiences suggest that the teacher assumes a more important role. The amount of time we recorded children engaging in book reading was related to later ability to talk about language on the word definition task ($r = .37$, $p < .05$); the amount of time teachers reported scheduling time for small group activities (including small group book reading) was linked to vocabulary ($r = .45$, $p < .05$) and to print skill ($r = .40$, $p < .40$); and the teacher's reported interest in fostering writing and using books in varied areas of the curriculum was related to vocabulary ($r = .36$, $p < .05$) and to story understanding ($r = .37$, $p < .05$). Thus, in contrast to the findings for three-year-olds, variables from the classrooms of four-year-olds that were related to kindergarten literacy predominantly require teacher input and direct involvement.

Teacher Agenda

As previously noted, teachers' agendas may have many sources (e.g., cultural, pedagogical) and they influence teacher–child interaction throughout the day. An example of the importance of variations in teachers' orientations to engaging children comes from our examination of how teachers read and discuss books with children. Group book reading events were videotaped in 25 classrooms. The reading of one book was transcribed in each room and coded for the general content of comments (e.g., analytical, describing pictures, controlling behavior), for the identity of the speakers (child or teacher), and for whether or not the comment was linked to previous or subsequent utterances (i.e., was the comment a response to a question or a request for a response?). Comments also were coded for whether they occurred while the book was being read or before or after it was completed (see Dickinson, 1992).

Consistent with previous research (Dickinson & Keebler, 1989), we found that teachers adopt different styles of reading books. Some teachers see book reading as a time for performing books, for drawing children into story worlds; others use books as a starting point for discussions about language, the world, and children's experiences; and still others use them as a time to work on particular school-like skills such as recalling the order of events or remembering specific factual details. Thus, teachers have different goals for book reading and these agendas have a major impact on the overall way the activity is structured.

The overall manner in which teachers read the book we analyzed was not strongly related to our outcome measures, perhaps because teachers shift approaches depending on factors such as the familiarity and genre of the book and the general attentiveness of children. In contrast to the results from the global classification of book reading style, our analysis of the kinds of questions teachers asked showed very strong relationships between book reading and language development. Using regression analyses, we found that interactions that involved teachers and children talking about texts in an analytical fashion as books were read (i.e., not prior to or following the actual reading of the text) were very strongly associated with vocabulary development (R^2 = .51, $p < .0001$) and somewhat less strongly with reading comprehension (R^2 = .25, $p < .01$). Given that we also found patterns of relationship between other classroom measures and these same outcomes, we were concerned that those teachers who engaged in analytical talk during book reading might also be the teachers who foster language growth throughout the day. Therefore, we constructed regression models that statistically controlled for the other variables that independently correlated with our outcomes to ensure that our assessment of the effects of book reading was not actually measuring these effects. After we controlled for these other aspects of classrooms, we found that child-involved analytical talk still was strongly associated with vocabulary development ($p < .01$). The relationship between book reading and story comprehension did not prove to be so clear. After we controlled for other aspects of the classroom program, the book reading variable no longer was significantly related to children's reading comprehension ability.

SUMMARY

It is clear from our data that children's experiences in preschool are related to emerging language and literacy skills at the end of kindergarten. The patterns of effects can be thought of as reflecting the interaction of the variables previously outlined (identity of speaker, activity type, teacher agenda). Correlations between classroom experience and language and literacy revealed that younger children who played with peers engaged in more pretending and that this type of activity was strongly linked to subsequent development. Four-year-olds who were involved in more book reading and other varied literacy-related activities and in book reading events in which teachers engaged in child-involved analytic talk showed stronger performance on our battery of kindergarten measures.

IMPLICATIONS FOR PRACTICE

Our data indicate that specific kinds of classroom experiences of low-income children during the preschool years can have a beneficial impact on their language and literacy development, effects that are observable a year or more after children have left those rooms. Our results point to the importance of particular kinds of classroom experiences, not simply the presence or absence of the opportunity to attend preschool. Examination of these effects points to the fact that we must take into consideration factors that condition the type of interactions in which children engage.

Teachers must consider whether children are talking with adults or peers, because the content of children's talk is related to the identity of their interactant. Furthermore, three-year-olds who spent more time talking with other children also spent more time engaged in pretend talk and these children did better on our measures of language and literacy development at the end of kindergarten. Although it is tempting to interpret this finding as indicating that classrooms in which our children were encouraged to engage in considerable amounts of pretend play caused them to develop stronger early literacy skills, our correlational data cannot support this interpretation. Indeed, we suspect that these correlations indicate that children who engaged in more pretending at age three were those with stronger linguistic skills, possibly because they had early home environments that were especially supportive of literacy and pretending. Whatever the ultimate explanation for this correlation, our results indicate that allowing children to interact with other children is very likely to result in pretend talk and that such interactions are linked to development of literacy-related skills.

Activity type, a third variable that is inextricably tied to conversational partners and agenda, also plays a vital role in shaping children's interactional experiences. Book reading and pretending are two important kinds of activities whose occurrence teachers control by virtue of scheduling decisions. Similarly, by planning varied activities involving small groups and including print (writing, dictating stories, reading varied materials), teachers can structure sessions that benefit children's emerging literacy skills.

Teachers have enormous influence over the shape of interactions with children, and the direction in which a teacher moves a conversation is heavily influenced by his or her immediate goals. To an extent these goals reflect structural factors such as whether the teacher's role is that of the circulating "overseer" of activities or the person in charge of directing a particular activity. However, teacher agendas also can vary within the same interactional setting. For a variety of reasons including book-related factors such as genre, familiarity, and personal preference, teachers vary in how they read books with children. This variability has important consequences. The predilection to engage children in interactive discussions about the meaning of stories and words is strongly linked to vocabulary development and somewhat less clearly to story comprehension.

Finally, children's developmental levels need to be taken into consideration. Three- and four-year-olds are at quite different points in development of language abilities and we are finding different patterns of correlations that suggest that these developmental differences are important. It appears that the more child-directed free play type activities may be of most benefit to the younger children whereas greater teacher input and small and large group activities that provide for rich language use may be of greater importance for older children.

In this chapter I have attempted to provide a framework for guiding teachers' thinking about the language environment. Thoughtful teachers will find many ways to extend it (see the appendix for a list of ideas). Where possible I provided data to support my contentions, but it is important to bear in mind three facts when considering this data: (1) these results come from a relatively small sample, a sample that includes only half of the 80 children in our entire sample; (2) many of the analyses are at a relatively early stage of refinement; and (3) our data reflect results from a study using children with normally developing language skills. Our suggestions related to development need to be examined by researchers and practitioners working with children with varying kinds of language delays to determine whether and how they might apply.

NOTES

This research was supported by grants from the Spencer Foundation and the Agency for Children, Youth and Families through a grant from project Head Start. I gratefully thank both for their support. I also thank Petra Nicholson for her many hours of work collecting, organizing, and analyzing data.

1. For details regarding tests and scoring procedures write to Patton Tabors, Larsen Hall, Third Floor, Harvard Graduate School of Education, Cambridge, MA 02138.

REFERENCES

Chafe, W. (1985). Linguistic differences produced by differences between speaking and writing. In D. R. Olson, N. Torrance, & A. Hildyard (Eds.), *Literacy, language and learning: The nature and consequences of reading and writing* (pp. 105–123). New York: Cambridge University Press.

De Temple, J., & Beals, D. E. (1991). Family talk: Sources of support for the development of decontextualized language skills. *Journal of Research in Childhood Education, 6,* 11–19.

Dickinson, D. K. (1987). Oral language, literacy skills and response to literature. In J. Squire (Ed.), *The dynamics of language learning: Research in the language arts* (pp. 147–183). Urbana, IL: National Council of Teachers of English.

Dickinson, D. K. (1991). Teacher stance and setting: Constraints on conversation in preschools. In A. McCabe & C. Peterson (Eds.), *Developing narrative structure* (pp. 255–302). Hillsdale, NJ: Lawrence Erlbaum.

Dickinson, D. K. (1992). Long-term effects of teacher-child discussions of books on low-income children's vocabulary and story understanding. In B. deBaryshe (Chair), *Emergent reading and book reading.* Symposium presented at the Human Development Conference, Atlanta, GA.

Dickinson, D. K., & McCabe, A. (1991). A social interactionist account of language and literacy development. In J. Kavanaugh (Ed.), *The language continuum.* Parkton, MD: The York Press.

Dickinson, D. K., & Keebler, R. (1989). Variation in preschool teachers' book reading styles. *Discourse Processes, 12,* 353–376.

Dickinson, D. K., & Smith, M. (1991). Preschool talk: Patterns of teacher–child interaction in early childhood classrooms. *Journal of Research in Childhood Education, 6,* 20–29.

Dickinson, D. K., & Tabors, P. (1991). Early literacy: Linkages between home, school, and literacy achievement at age five. *Journal of Research in Childhood Education, 6,* 30–46.

Heath, S. B. (1986). Separating "things of imagination" from life: Learning to read and write. In W. Teale & E. Sulzby (Eds.), *Emergent literacy: Writing and reading* (pp. 156–172). Norwood, NJ: Ablex.

Michaels, S. (1991). The dismantling of narrative. In A. McCabe & C. Peterson (Eds.), *Developing narrative structure* (pp. 303–355). Hillsdale, NJ: Lawrence Erlbaum.

Minami, M., & McCabe, A. (1991). *Haiku* as a discourse regulation device: A stanza analysis of Japanese children's personal narratives. *Language in Society, 20,* 577–600.

Snow, C. E., Cancino, H., Gonzalez, P., & Shriberg, E. (1989). Giving formal defi-
    nitions: An oral language correlate of school literacy. In D. Bloome (Ed.),
    Classrooms and literacy (pp. 233–249). Norwood, NJ: Ablex.
Torrance, N., & Olson, D. R. (1985). Oral and literate competencies in the early
    school years. In D. R. Olson, N. Torrance, & A. Hildyard (Eds.), *Literacy and
    language learning* (pp. 256–284). New York: Cambridge University Press.

APPENDIX

Recommendations for Practice

The following is a list of suggestions for classroom practices likely to foster development of language and literacy abilities of young children. All are based on prior research—some of it is work that we have done and reported within the chapter, and some has been done by other researchers.

OBJECTIVE: INCREASE OPPORTUNITIES FOR EXTENDED TALK ABOUT TOPICS THAT REQUIRE COMMUNICATION OF NEW INFORMATION

1. **Put language development on the teacher's agenda at all times**
   Possible strategies:

   a. Avoid overuse of predictable topics such as colors, counting; don't be afraid of complex topics (e.g., machinery, shadows, death)

   b. Be aware of comments that close out child comments (e.g., mechanical responses such as "isn't that nice?")

   c. Strive to encourage children to evaluate experiences, to speculate about reasons for events, to predict outcomes; this is relatively easy with small groups and when working with a challenging curriculum

   d. Support children's efforts to communicate complex thoughts (e.g., wait patiently, suggest words as needed)

   e. Encourage multiple forms of symbolization and make linkages among them (e.g., begin with painting and extend into storytelling or drama)

   f. Tell personal stories; ask questions about things that interest you; acknowledge uncertainty and model efforts to learn answers to your questions

2. **Plan for teacher availability during free play times**
   Possible strategies:

   a. Keep one teacher stationary during activity times (leading activities or extending ongoing activity—especially valuable with small groups)

   b. Have a "Personal Experiences" center in the classroom where a teacher is positioned during a portion of choice times for hearing important personal events and recording them

   c. Plan art or drama activities and through them draw children into discussions about personal experiences or begin with personal experiences and build curriculum from them

   d. Have area for experimenting with intriguing machines (e.g., broken typewriter, door knobs, zippers, etc.; encourage children to explain how they work; encourage sharing of explanations in small groups)

    e. Have small groups of children report on activities or display products; help them explain how they did them

3. **Plan for teacher availability during snack and meal times**
(Requires considerable planning and preparation ahead of time)
Possible strategies:

    a. Allow children to control conversational topics

    b. Encourage talk about personal experiences

    c. Encourage curiosity questions (e.g., about food—what it is made of, where it comes from, how it helps your body, etc.)

4. **Make books a central part of the language enhancement program**
Possible strategies:

    a. Be aware of *how* you read and discuss books; allow children opportunities to ask questions and comment on stories; strive to ask "how" and "why" questions but beware of losing the story line—don't kill the story with talk

    b. Reread stories and push for deeper understandings

    c. Encourage children to read familiar books with you

    d. Make familiar books available in the room for use in free time

    e. Build books into integrated units and plan activities that extend themes (e.g., drama, songs, art)

    f. Provide props to encourage children to enact the story when playing alone

    g. Have favorite books on tape and encourage children to listen to the tapes while looking at the books

    h. Extend units with library books; take children with you as you check out books for classroom use

5. **Structure times for extended talk about personal experiences**
Possible strategies:

    a. When children first arrive have one teacher available for routine sharing of recent events; be available to parent and child (parent may help child); write these down for later discussion

    b. At the end of the day have time for children to discuss the day (e.g., successes, problems, memories); for young children have chart with plan for day available as memory aid (have picture clues to help)

    c. Help individuals and small or full groups make tape recordings of favorite stories; encourage children to listen to tapes

6. **Encourage rich pretending among children**
   Possible strategies:

   a. Provide sufficiently long periods of time to allow children to develop complex pretend play

   b. Provide props that encourage the linking of dramatic play to ongoing units or favorite books

   c. Provide props that support use of familiar scripts (e.g., restaurant, house, grocery store); especially useful for younger children

   d. Change props and organization periodically to maintain interest levels

7. **Encourage families to help extend activities you initiate**
   Possible strategies:

   a. Loan copies of currently favorite books and encourage parents to tell you of their experiences reading them with their children

   b. Tell parents the title of their child's favorite books and encourage use of the library to get a copy of that book or similar books

   c. Tell parents of current units; suggest ways to extend them

NOTE

These suggestions were developed with the assistance of Miriam Smith. I would be interested in hearing from teachers or researchers who have experimented with some of these ideas and want to share their findings with me. Write to me at Education Department, Clark University, 950 Main St., Worcester, MA 01610.

NAME INDEX

Note: Bold numbers refer to the reference section at the end of each chapter.

Vihman, M., 150, **162**
Volterra, V., 23, 24, **42**

W

Waletsky, J., 89, 90, **103**
Warren, D., 43, **58**
Waterson, N., 55
Watson-Gegeo, K., 30, **42**
Wechsler, D., 66, **71**
Weinreich, U., 22, **42**
Weitzner-Lin, B., 136, 139, 140, **148,**
    149, **160**
Wellman, H., 75, 79, 80, **87**
Wells, G., 55, 105, 106, **119**
Westby, C., 107, 110, 112, **119,** 136,
    139, **148**
Whitehurst, G., 175, **184**
Whiten, A., 77, **85**
Wiebe, J., 91, **104**

Wiig, E., 55
Wimmer, H., 76, 80, **87**
Wolf, D., 110, **119**
Wolf, S., 170, **184**
Wong-Fillmore, L., 149, 150, 152, 159,
    162
Woodruff, G., 75, **87**
Woolley, J., 79, **87**
Wu, H., 175, **182**

Y

Yaniv, I., 79, **87**
Yirmiya, N., 93, **104**
Yoder, D., 106, **119**

Z

Zentella, A., 27, 28, 29, 39, **42**

SUBJECT INDEX

A

African-American culture, 156
Age:
  influence on language and literacy,
    192, 193, 196
  and teacher expectations, 192
  three- vs. four-year-olds, 192, 193,
    196
Agendas (*see also* Teacher agendas),
  186, 191–92, 194–95
Analytic intervention, 149, 150
  breaking down gestalt units, 159
  slot filling, 159
Analytic learner (*see also* Learners),
  156, 157, 158
Autism, 8, 92–101, 151

B

Behaviorism, 72
Belief–desire psychology, 74

Bilingualism, 20–42
  abstract structures vs.
    linguistic practice, 26
  balanced, 26
  benefits of, 22
  in children, 21–42
  code separation, 24, 25, 26
  in established speech
    communities, 23
  interference (*see* Bilingualism, lan-
    guage mixing)
  language mixing, 23, 24, 25, 26
  vs. monolingual acquisition, 25
  one vs. two language systems, 24,
    25, 26
  role of language input (*see also* Lan-
    guage input), 22, 25, 26, 32
  simultaneous acquisition of lan-
    guages, 22, 24
  in situations of conflict, 23
  studies using self reports, 24, 25,
    38
  syntactic development, 24